BY THE SAME AUTHOR

Conquering Cancer

Decision Making

Decision-Making

The Modern Doctor's Dilemma

Reflections on the Art of Medicine

Lucien Israël, M.D.

Translated from the French
by Mary Feeney

Random House
New York

 Published in the United States by Random House, Inc., New York and simultaneously in Canada by Random House of Canada Limited, Toronto. Originally published in France as *La Décision Médicale: Essai sur l'art de la médecine* by Calmann-Lévy, Paris.

Library of Congress Cataloging in Publication Data

Israël, Lucien.
Decision-making—the modern doctor's dilemma.

Translation of: La décision médicale.
Bibliography: p.
1. Medicine—Philosophy. 2. Medicine—Decision making. 3. Medical logic. I. Title.
R723.18413 616'.001 81-48286
ISBN 0-394-51528-5 AACR2

Manufactured in the United States of America

98765432

FIRST EDITION

To Danielle, Dominique, Guillaume

More facts are true than can be proved.

—GÖDEL

Life is short, art is long, events are fleeting,
experience is deceptive, judgement is difficult.

—HIPPOCRATUS

Foreword

The world's men and women collectively make and experience history, scrutinize the past, envision the future, engage in armed conflict. But when sickness strikes them or their loved ones, they are suddenly reduced to the dimensions of their own short life on this earth. For this reason the status of medicine has always been ambiguous and always will be. When we are healthy, we ridicule doctors. We begrudge them their failures, which are merely the failure of the individual in the context of the species. But when we are in a physician's care, we transfer to him the belief, the love, the veneration that medicine's powerful magic inspires. And then, predictably enough, society comes into the picture, legislating, setting prices, ordering expenditures, planning, establishing the medical-school curriculum.

The sociology of medicine, however little it has been studied, is neither my subject nor my specialty; nor is epistemology. In the natural course of events, however, the physician inevitably asks himself questions about his work, its methods and consequences, its imperfections and their remedies, as well as the cultural trends molding his image and the demands made on him. The last few decades have witnessed a considerable change in the powers of medicine. Neither the physician, the epistemologist, nor the public has gauged its meaning.

Until the end of the nineteenth century, the implicit demand on the doctor was to offer not a cure but a prognosis. The successful physician was one who could tell if the patient would recover. By interpreting certain signs, he could read the immediate future. Other than that, he was essentially expected to comfort the sick. The surgeon alone was a man of action. Prescribing an operation was for a long time the only real choice available to medicine. Subsequently, following the natural tendency toward refining the prognosis, the diagnostician came to the fore with advances in nosology gleaned from the examination of clinical and postmortem data. The mark of the outstanding physician was an inclination to classify; when faced with an apparently unclear situation, he was able to identify a disease and predict its course, though without intervening. Today doctors still have the intellectual "game" of making a diagnosis as soon as possible without recourse to exterior means. And they are still apt to be mistaken. However, considerable advances in biological diagnosis and the visualization of the internal organs have reduced both the margins of error and the proportion of art in medicine. Although there is still talk of flair, of intuition, meaning that the whole spectrum of possibilities is sometimes examined by something other than a conscious, systematic exploration, that is well behind us now; we teach our medical students to leave nothing to chance, to be conscientious workmen, to search for the evidence they need to proceed to the next step.

Does this mean that the medical artist has watched the range of his talent shrink, then vanish in the face of technology? It would be closer to the truth to say that the art I am talking about is needed in a different place. It has little part to play in prognosis or diagnosis any more. On the other hand, it is vitally important in the domain of therapeutics—a strange statement, but one easily justified.

Within the past thirty years, medical science has been totally transformed by antibiotics, hormones, immunosuppressants, anti-inflammatory and anti-cancer drugs, not to mention impressive advances in surgery and reanimation. In these thirty years, the physician's role has changed from one of botanical contemplation to one of commando action. Medicine can now dissect complex biological mechanisms, can block the development of structural and biochemical disorders by intervening at the molecular level. Soothsaying, in short, has yielded to engineering. And, quite naturally, more is asked of the physician today than ever before. People have quickly gotten accustomed to the breadth of medicine's powers; now these powers simply seem too limited, too flawed. Their very effectiveness allows us to propose a new classification of disease, reflecting medicine's current situation and powers of healing.

Most diseases are spontaneously curable. They must be watched for complications, and treatment to alleviate discomfort may be indicated. A more intensive therapeutic program may also cut the disease short. Each case dictates its own treatment. There are also diseases that used to be dangerous which are now almost always curable with adequate treatment. Here the error is either misdiagnosing the disease or prescribing the wrong treatment, both of which are very rare occurrences. The medical decisions in these cases fall within the realm of certainty. Improved treatments may of course still be found, but the real danger has been eliminated.

On the other hand, we can still point to two instances in which medicine always falls short: incurable diseases that destroy vital functions, such as massive cerebral hemorrhage; and incurable but chronic diseases such as asthma or arthritis. Treatment for discomfort has improved, and it is now easier to keep the diseases from spreading. But the diseases themselves cannot be arrested.

Finally, a new area has opened up: the treatment of diseases that in the past were always fatal but can now sometimes be cured or controlled: cancer, acute kidney failure, heart disease. In certain cases —providing the appropriate treatment is carried out in time, in adequate sequences, following specific guidelines—the survival rate has climbed from 0 percent to 20 percent, 50 percent, even 75 percent.

These statistics are at once reassuring and disturbing—reassuring in that they show our progress in mastering nature, but disturbing to the extent that they also illustrate our uncertainty regarding individual destiny. It should be kept in mind that these percentages are not static. The survival rate is steadily climbing, thanks to the ongoing efforts of all those in the field. I would like to add that the rate of success differs from one medical team to the next, one physician to the next, one strategy to the next.

Here we have a very specific area of medical endeavor. Day by day it grows in influence, yet its distinguishing characteristic is the uncertainty of its end results. There are two ways to optimize our performance in this field. Unlike many of my colleagues, I do not find them mutually exclusive but rather complementary. The first is reducing uncertainty until it becomes certainty. By this I mean clinical research, a new and necessary tool of medicine, now experiencing its growing pains. Determining the powers and limits of research is crucial.

The second way to optimize our performance would be to apply advances in decision theory to medicine. Without really being aware of it, the physician has become a decision-maker, working under uncertainty. He is not playing an intelligent opponent, as he would be in Von Neumann and Morgenstern's classic game theory. The physician's opponent is nature, meaning a heightened degree of uncertainty. It is interesting to note that while the recent past has brought important advances in the theory of decision under uncertainty, and while uncertainty can now be expressed in mathematical terms—an impressive feat to a layman like me—the theory has been applied only in the fields of the military, economics and management. The various theoretical works I have consulted make no mention of the problems of decision in medicine, just as all of medical literature contains only a dozen or so references to decision theory.

This was my initial reason for undertaking this book. Only a tiny proportion of clinical observations can be used in the framework of a rigorous clinical methodology, as I will later explain. In the overwhelming majority of cases, the physician working in this field must decide on strategy case by case. Each patient is a new problem, with his or her own terrain, which includes the extent and stage of the disease and the amount of suffering involved. There are also the patient's specific demands, degree of awareness and assessment of tolerable secondary effects. These are just some of the things that must be taken into account in constructing a winning strategy that allows physician and patient to prevail over numerous insufficiently controlled or understood or even completely unknown factors.

These are the problems we face at the forefront of medicine, and no one ever taught us that this is how it would be.

It is hardly surprising, then, that physicians know little or nothing about decision analysis. Many of my students seem to think that a given situation automatically implies a stereotyped therapeutic response. Some of them see a choice between two or three methods of treatment. Few of them realize there are perhaps twenty different "plays" worth trying. And not one of them has ever heard of decision trees, subjective probability, coherence comparability, utilities, multicriteria choices.

I am not the one to cast the first stone, since my own acquaintance with decision theory is unfortunately recent. But in addition to this particular shortcoming, there are other gaps in medical knowledge. Too many patients are treated in terms of choices whose rationale is difficult to grasp, decisions only their maker can justify. Often not even the minimum rules that should govern decision-making are present, and instinct reigns. Sometimes it triumphs, but it is far from the safest way to proceed.

It therefore struck me that it would be useful to point out this problem, call it to the attention of those physicians and mathematicians whose mutual concern it ought to be, and consider the possibility of resultant changes in the medical curriculum.

The first thing decision experts tell us is that a decision should not be approached until its consequences have been defined. Thanks to this bit of wisdom I clearly saw (for the first time, I must admit) that there is no written code of medical ethics; there are no courses in medical ethics in our curriculum, and each physician must in the course of his professional life come up with his own set of ethics and consider the consequences of his practice. This difficult question is one I will have to examine in some detail; it is part and parcel of the first problem I discuss.

It is obvious that the physician must have the most complete information, must refer to a clearly defined value system and a knowledge of consequences, deduce from them precise objectives, and then elaborate an inspired strategy for meeting those objectives. And all this has to be done in the face of great uncertainty. Striving toward this goal is the least the physician can do, since he has chosen to be the guardian and repository of what his fellow human beings hold most precious: their health and their trust. In return, the least society can do is uphold the moral stature of those on whom it confers such a responsibility, rather than regard them as purveyors of some kind of product.

It is not a question of striking a bargain, however. Out of respect for others and for themselves, physicians are obliged to combine all the available resources of science and art, and place them at the disposal of every patient. They must also steer those unsuited for medicine toward other careers.

Beyond the implicit obligation to be above reproach and to operate on the only acceptable level—that of excellence—some physicians have another mission: to chart out uncertain territory, innovate, imagine new strategies. They are the ones who are given the difficult or hopeless cases. They must mobilize their resources of intellect and logic in order to overcome the unknown in nature. In this struggle they are supported to some extent by the new tool I have already mentioned, clinical research. If they wish, they may also have the use of the tools forged by decision theorists.

I hope to show in this book how the diverse aspects of medicine fit together. It will become evident, I think, that the medical arts are not a vestige of the dark ages, liable to be replaced by computers. The problem our societies face is rather how to recruit and train talented artists if medicine is to be one day acknowledged as a high, noble and strictly essential calling.

Contents

DECISION MAKING

CHAPTER I

On Certain Nontherapeutic Dimensions of Medicine

BEFORE REACHING the point at which clinical decisions must be made, the physician is more or less implicitly forced to go through a series of evaluations and calculations whose conclusions influence his subsequent commitment to the case and the treatment he prescribes. It is therefore important to examine this process to help clarify the nature of medical practice. These are the factors the physician must take into account:

I *Is Disease Present?*

This is probably one of the hardest decisions for the doctor to make. Often a patient erroneously takes certain sensations or changes in bodily function for signs of serious illness, while just as frequently the real symptoms of a disease are ignored, sometimes by the same person. The patient is not objective by definition or position, nor is he detached from what is happening to him. His emotions affect, may even create, his symptoms. How well or poorly informed he is, his past or present circumstances, influence the way he pictures his condition, determine the level of his fears and thus the importance he gives to each of the various phenomena he experiences.There are occasional cases of hypochondria, obsessive fixations on sensations that are not observably pathological. Sometimes the power of suggestion comes into play: a patient complaining of a nagging sore throat, for example, has a friend who was just operated on for cancer of the larynx. Some types of muscle spasm have no pathological origin. In the same way, the aging process produces very different symptoms in different people.

Insidious diseases, however, certainly do exist, and their stealthy development can be unmasked only with the help of tedious, restrictive, even "invasive" (as our jargon has it) testing, and the tests sometimes carry a certain risk.

Finally, there are unidentified diseases with uncharacteristic symptoms which it is all too easy to attribute to the patient's imagination or impressionable character.

Thus the physician must know when to withhold any drastic measures, which might among other things wrongly convince the patient that he is "sick." At the same time, a doctor must be wary of reassuring a patient too quickly; he must neither encourage the patient's natural optimism nor stir up his subconscious terror.

Yet the physician we are talking about is not a logical machine but a creature of flesh and blood just like the patient. Dr. Portes, a former president of France's Ordre des Médecins (national medical association), defined the relationship of doctor and patient as the meeting point of trust on the one hand, conscience on the other. So be it. It is also a meeting of two ways of looking at the world, which can mean differences in education, moral outlook, opinions, frustrations. This gives one some idea of how highly demanding the medical profession is, and rightly so, since a physician should be able to put aside all the elements of his personal equation and accept those of the person he is working with to form a perfectly objective image of the case at hand. This assumes the physician has given sufficient thought to how we define the norm and the acceptable range of variations to be able to decide if the patient has consulted him because he is sick or because he is concerned for the wrong reason. The physician's skill and knowledge must be up to the task in situations so varied that they defy cataloguing. Here I might note that although systematic and thorough examination and testing could eliminate the chance of error, that is no solution, since the cost and the risks involved would be exorbitant. Only an heuristic approach would favor such a position, but it is far from the only approach. Many different disciplines can contribute to increasing the proportion of logic a medical decision contains. But at the same time, it is impossible to eliminate completely the heuristic attitude inherent in any choice.

Are There Symptoms of Serious Illness?

After the doctor has determined that disease is indeed present, he must decide whether it is an illness that will clear up spontaneously in a few days; or an illness that is no longer serious because it now responds to a simple, accepted treatment; or one of those cases that is never given a name but simply disappears, to everyone's relief; or a complaint whose symptoms should not be "cooled down," since this might cover up the signs of a serious disorder. This is often a delicate choice. To put it in another way: How far should the physician go with diagnostic procedures that are costly in terms of time, undesirable side effects, even risk to the patient?

It is quite evident that in addition to skill, experience and acuity of observation, a practitioner's character plays a part in the decision-making process: his self-confidence or lack of it, his optimistic or pessimistic cast of mind, as well as perhaps his memory of a recent success or failure. The only solution is total modesty—not to hesitate to recognize one's perplexity, to admit it and to solicit a knowledgeable colleague's opinion —plus a permanent effort to improve, which may help first to attenuate, then to eliminate interfering traits and sharpen the indispensable sixth sense.

Should Treatment Be Undertaken?

This question comes up if the disease will cure itself without treatment, or if it is incurable. But even then there is no simple answer. How can we be so cruel as to refuse treatment to someone whose only hope is centered on all-powerful medical technology? On the other hand, in the case of a benign, self-curing infection, can we refuse to respond to suffering with a prescription when the medicine represents to the patient both his health and the fact that he is now under someone else's care?

It would be nice if we could explain to every patient that his fever, stomach problems, insomnia, will clear up spontaneously. It would be nice if patients understood, and they would if only we all achieved maturity. Unfortunately we do not, so medical decision-making hinges on how sure the doctor is in his estimation of the patient's independence. It is good to be able to tell someone, "Don't ask for outside help when there is nothing to fear. Accept the temporary discomfort. Even without medication, your illness will leave no trace. The same thing will happen again in your lifetime, without hindering or shortening it." But sometimes this advice falls on deaf ears. The patient will then consult other doctors and come to resent what he eventually remembers as a sadistic refusal to treat him.

But here again the choice does not depend exclusively on the patient's personality. What kind of person is the doctor making the decision: independent, fretful, aggressive?

Telling the Truth

The problem of whether or not to tell a patient the truth is essentially connected to cases of serious illness or diseases the public considers fatal, such as cancer. When I discussed truthfulness in an earlier work,* certain critics in the United States objected to the nuances I allowed for, while many European readers and doctors thought I was too strongly in favor of telling the truth.

Because my subject here is decision-making, I will limit myself to saying only that telling the whole truth about diagnosis and prognosis is a service to some patients and a disservice to others. Unless it becomes a matter of law—which to my mind would be a mistake—the physician should be allowed to decide when only part of the truth, or none of it, should best be told.

But once again, what kind of person is the doctor making the choice? A flawless judge of character? A fearless and dispassionate physician, determined to serve to the utmost? Or an ordinary person with repressed fears, superstitions, unconscious sadism or faith in the superiority of his own philosophical opinions?

A Few Other Decisions

A good many choices have to be made, explicitly or implicitly, before any medical advice is given. What, for instance, should the limits of abnormality be? How high a cholesterol or blood-pressure level is too high?

Some people are surprised to learn that there is no one answer to such questions. Age, heredity, morphology, sex, the

**Conquering Cancer,* Random House, 1978

presence of other abnormal factors influence the decision, so that the evaluation depends largely on the doctor's individual experience.

Should a practitioner consulted for a case of the flu show alarm at a weight problem and suggest evaluating and treating it? Should he ask the patient about his smoking habits, and if he smokes, advise him to quit, even if there are no obvious ill effects at the time of the examination? How many cancer patients have responded to my order to stop smoking with: "You're the first doctor who ever told me to." Should we ask about a family history of certain diseases, determine whether the patient belongs to a high-risk group and then suggest or prescribe follow-up procedures, even if that was not why the patient consulted us in the first place? Among a whole range of possible choices, there are two extremes: treating simply the disorder the patient originally came in for, or ordering a complete physical examination, including evaluations by various specialists. Another possibility would be to tell the patient what should be checked on in the near future, perhaps followed up by preventive measures, exploratory procedures or treatment.

Decisions like these are of course highly influenced by the kind of health-care situation in which the patient and physician meet, as well as the pressure society exerts in the financial area. The physician's personal philosophy and image of his practice are also very important.

Even before a therapy is established, then, the patient is embarking on an adventure, confronting a professional decision-maker who—sometimes within minutes—will examine a whole gamut of choices, reject certain strategies and adopt others, narrowing the range of future choices. These choices can lead to irreversible decisions without either the doctor or the patient being aware of it; both should be made to realize this. Complaining about medical power is not productive.

Medical power is a matter of fact. It is essentially based on knowledge, and denying it would lead to the emergence of powers dangerous in other ways. It *is* necessary, however, to analyze the breadth of medical power, its limits and dangers, the ways it is used, and to envision ways to eliminate potential abuses, retaining only the positive aspects. That is what this book is in part about.

CHAPTER II

The Dimensions of Therapeutic Uncertainty

I *Certainty and Uncertainty*

I have yet to be convinced that certainty ever exists in therapeutic situations. By "certainty" I mean that the prescribing physician is certain he knows all the consequences, both short- and long-term, of the treatment, which should be risk-free. If this were the case, the most complex medical problems would be merely a matter of linear programming, but in all likelihood we will never reach this point. Uncertainty, as we shall see, is part and parcel of the therapeutic decision with one important exception: cases where there is the certainty of failure if nothing is done and therefore of having nothing to lose in trying something.

It is not easy to describe the kind of uncertainty we are dealing with. As I understand it, the first kind of uncertainty mathematicians mastered was game theory against an intelligent opponent trying to win and using various tactics. In his famous zero-sum game theory, Von Neumann showed that it was possible to adopt a strategy likely to minimize losses and maximize gain, no matter how the opponent played. Arriving at such a strategy involves foreseeing all the opponent's possible tactics from the outset and calculating the results of different defensive plays.

The study of gamesmanship gave rise to a wealth of applications and fascinating writing on the subject, which is unfortunately of no help to doctors because, as I said before, doctors are not playing against an intelligent opponent determined to win according to certain rules, but against nature, which means a considerable body of laws of causality intertwined in a practically infinite network. Every move a doctor makes has unintentional and potentially hazardous consequences. However, in measuring the consequences of all possible courses of treatment and the possible results of each treatment, doctors are dealing with uncertainty that can be expressed in terms of mathematical probability, and there has already been a great deal of mathematical discussion of the subject. In certain situations of extreme uncertainty, when the number of possible outcomes is incalculable and their probability unknown, mathematical theory is as yet of little help. A doctor treating serious illness is almost always caught between these two dimensions of uncertainty. Indeed, the reason some diseases are serious is precisely because the conditions for controlling them are inadequately understood.

Uncertainty About Causes

The causes of certain severe diseases, such as tetanus or rabies, have already been discovered. Even so, many pathogens remain unidentified, and new infectious diseases continue to appear (for example, Legionnaire's Disease). It is virtually certain that most syndromes of unknown origin are caused by viruses, but the viruses have not yet been identified.

In the realm of diseases probably unrelated to infection, a great deal of uncertainty remains. What causes arthritis, kidney disease, certain kinds of emphysema in the young, psoriasis? And what causes cancer? This is where we fully appreciate not only how vast but also how complex the task at hand is. We know that several unrelated factors probably play a role before cancer starts developing: genetic predisposition, the presence of carcinogens, radiation, a virus, a passing immunological weakness, but when it comes to cancer in human beings, a spontaneous disease occurring in a complex environment, we are not close to identifying the cause or causes.

This does not mean that doctors should be discouraged about treating cancer; they never have been before. The entire history of medicine can be summed up as a series of more or less successful attempts to control, if not cure, diseases of unknown origin. A very good example is what has been happening in the treatment of leukemia over the last twenty years. Of course, cancer specialists construct theories on the causes of the diseases they treat and test them against facts (when they are lucky enough to be objective) or else vehemently defend their theories when they contend that "logic" is a substitute for scientific knowledge. But in the final analysis, theories evolve, replace others and disappear, while medicine's concrete powers continue to grow steadily. Sometimes the theories are nothing new. Colchicine helped relieve gout, for example, long before the cause of the disease was known.

There can be no doubt, however, that in many cases knowing the cause of a disease would make everything infinitely easier. Yet even now causes elude us, and the resulting level of uncertainty means the physician proceeds haltingly, using empirically based strategies against the unknown in nature.

Uncertainty About the Mechanisms of Disease

In addition to all that has just been said, identifying the cause of a disease does not tell us anything about how it works to produce the disorders we observe. How does staphylococcus eventually produce an abscess of the lung? How does alcohol cause the lesions we observe in cirrhosis of the liver? Questions like these have to do with what medicine calls pathogenesis. Today we know that molecular and cellular biology, enzymology, immunology, and genetics can provide partial answers. Often investigation at the proper level is impossible for lack of the necessary technology, in which case doctors are unable to develop their clinical counterattack. Surefire strategies cannot be formulated when we do not know what we are fighting. On the other hand, sometimes the pathogenic process has been elucidated—a chronic inflammation, allergy, autoimmunity—while the cause is still unknown. Doctors then try a synthetic approach, treating similar disorders with similar means, even though they know a great disparity in the causes of the diseases may one day be revealed. This approach has had startling success in some instances, none at all in others.

Uncertainty About the Importance of Individual Differences

Here we enter into a crucial debate. As far back as Hippocrates, medical men made a careful distinction among different human temperaments, and ever since there have been numerous attempts to determine which character types are susceptible to certain diseases or best equipped to fight them. We are now discovering, through the work of the French biologist Dausset, that there are genetic groups determined by the presence or absence of various combinations of the genes carrying biological identity. Within these groups the probable occurrence of certain diseases is more likely than it is in a random sample of the population. This is doubtless the beginning of a great biological and medical adventure. If genetic differences govern the occurrence of nonhereditary diseases, we can expect to be able eventually to chart an individual's chances of contracting one disease or another, which would represent a major advance in preventive and diagnostic medicine.

We should also expect to learn more about individual resistance to a particular disease, why in one case breast cancer spreads so rapidly while in another it remains localized for six years. Differences in the development of cancer are of course observable only after the fact, when a patient tells us she first noticed an ulcerated tumor in one of her breasts several years earlier. We can then adopt a strategy appropriate to the slow spread of the disease. But when cancer is discovered in its earliest stages, we do not have the benefit of such knowledge. Will it develop rapidly or slowly? Should we simply back up the body's natural defenses, if possible, or should we attempt to destroy the cancer by medical means? If we also knew the biological nature of the differences between the two groups, it might become possible to make use of the distinction to turn highly invasive cases into slowly developing ones. But today we must still either make indirect evaluations of how a disease will progress or construct our strategies without any information at all.

Uncertainty About the Dangers of Drugs

This is usually not a major problem, since the probabilities of dangerous side effects can be clearly calculated in the vast majority of cases. Before any pharmaceutical product comes into general use, it undergoes a prolonged testing period, providing us with information about the frequency of risk, allergic reaction, or interference with kidney or liver function, and how serious each might be. It is then possible to decide in each individual case if it is worth running the risk, if other drugs might be used and whether or not the undesirable side effects could be minimized or offset. Nevertheless, the inventory of possible dangers can never be exhaustive, and every program of treatment carries an element of risk. It may be linked to a drug or to anesthesia, a testing procedure or surgery. The doctor knows what it is and plans around it.

Uncertainty About What Happens to Drugs

Our uncertainty about how medications work is all the greater because of the impressive variations we observe from one patient to the next in terms of biological reaction to drugs. A short while ago, we did not even know where in the body drugs usually ended up. Only the recent developments in pharmacokinetics, the study of what happens to drugs inside the human body, have shown us what happens to some—certainly not all—drugs when they enter the human body, which organs they affect, how long they stay there, how quickly they are eliminated, and even the by-products of their use or breakdown within the body. Our information is still far from complete. Nor do we know how therapeutic agents work. It was not until very recently that we learned something about how aspirin and certain antibiotics work, drugs that were known to be effective and therefore dispensed haphazardly, considering how little we knew about how and where they work.

The uncertainty about drugs is even more acute than this. Not every individual reacts the same way on the molecular level. There are differences in the breakdown and elimination of a drug, and in the distribution and effects of a drug's various derivatives or residues. Some years ago, it was determined that certain patients absorbed and eliminated isoniazid, an antibiotic used against tuberculosis, three times faster than others. Treating them with the usual doses of antibiotics was a failure. In this instance, uncertainty has disappeared. A simple test now determines which patients assimilate the drug rapidly, and their dosage is adjusted accordingly. Still, this is far from the case for all drugs now in use; there is still a good deal of risk involved when we prescribe drugs, even when we are familiar with how they work.

And that is not all. The disease's lesions themselves can respond very differently to treatment. Chemotherapy for cancer often runs up against this stumbling block: some cancer cells are able through mutation to break down a drug or prevent it from penetrating their membranes. But how many resisting cells are there in a tumor, and how many are simultaneously resistant to several drugs? We have no direct way of finding out. In cases like this, the knowledge of the risk of resistance, which can be expressed in terms of probability but not directly measured, must have a direct effect on the choice of treatment.

Medications can also interact with one another. Any relatively severe pathological disorder is almost sure to involve treatment with more than one medication. The disease must be attacked, but at the same time there may be a need to alleviate pain, induce sleep, compensate for kidney malfunction, and so forth. Pharmacologists have learned, for example, that phenobarbital in conjunction with the liver activates the breakdown of any other drugs administered, with variations from one patient to the next. In the future we will either have to test all the combinations of medication in every patient before beginning a program of treatment, or else we will have to learn to make decisions under uncertainty which can be expressed in terms of probability. We can then evaluate the results of our decisions and make better ones the next time.

Finally there are receptors, molecules either on the cell surface or in cell matter that collect the body's circulating products, such as hormones. Secreted by the endocrine glands, hormones simply pass through cells without receptors for them but act on cells that do have receptors. Some types of cancer are hormonodependent—that is, their cells have receptors for certain hormones, though this may vary from cell to cell and from one part of the tumor to another. This feature has provided a very important direction for treatment in certain types of breast cancer; the doctor can prescribe a suppressant for the hormone to which the cancer is linked. Yet this kind of knowledge leads only to uncertainty on a more detailed level. In the case of breast cancer alone, receptors have been found for such widely different hormones as estrogen, progesterone, testosterone, cortisone, prolactin, insulin. Some of them encourage the growth of cancer cells with receptors for them; others inhibit it. It is very difficult, and in practice often impossible, to know how receptors are distributed when cancer recurs internally. On the other hand, one cannot rule out hormone therapy when it might be of use. What is the best way to maximize its advantages with a minimum of "losses"?

It so happens that the receptors for morphine found in certain nerve cells led researchers to theorize that the human body must secrete a substance similar to the drug. The result was the recent, epoch-making discovery of endorphins, a group of amino acids in the brain that act as natural pain suppressants or opiates of the body. But there are also receptors for certain derivatives of tranquilizers and perhaps for alcohol, which seem to explain some types of chemical addiction. Could there also be receptors for various medications? If so, one thing is certain: they do not occur in every individual in the same way, one more reason certainty is hard to come by in this area.

This list of reasons for uncertainty in clinical situations is far from complete. In discussing the subject, I have tried to give some idea of the scope of the problem to those who imagine that the practice of medicine means merely following a formula mechanically once a disease has been typed, if not identified. In certain extreme cases this may be true. But for the most part, and especially in treating serious illness, uncertainty predominates, and treatment means gambling against nature.

As a result, some well-meaning research scientists working in laboratories wonder if it wouldn't be better to hold off treatment until they discover the causes and workings of the diseases. Before examining what is happening in the medical field, meaning the specific, concrete problems of decision-making and how they are solved, it seems to me essential to state the physician's point of view as opposed to the laboratory researcher's. I will also explain why there are people who in the face of so much uncertainty agree to make decisions and take action in such a difficult domain.

CHAPTER III

Medicine as an Autonomous Discipline

THE MAJOR REASON for the existence of medicine as we know it is, quite obviously, human suffering. We mortals never have been and never will be resigned to letting the guardians of organized, formalized knowledge tell us when and how to find remedies for our illnesses. Many "pure" scientists have already declared that trying to treat cancer is futile until they determine the cause of various types of cancer and deduce the appropriate treatment. Many laboratory researchers in immunology hold that we do not know enough about disorders of the immunological system to be able to treat them or even to try to arrest their natural development.

To answer this point of view, it is not necessary to point to the host of people who expect something to be done for them here and now. A "pure" scientist need only experience illness himself in order to realize (sometimes to his irritation) how naive his attitude is. Suddenly he no longer demands that the rules of logic be applied to his cure. He may not even demand a "cure," but only that he be given longer to live (if the disease is life-threatening). When it is a matter of his own body, the same person who winced at medicine's crude methods expects and accepts whatever treatment the medical arts can provide.

It is easy to predict that the demand for medicine will never abate, just as uncertainty will never completely disappear from the clinical picture. It is even evident that the demand for medical help is steadily growing, that people are less and less willing to accept the "injustice" of illness, the "outrage" of death or even the weakening of physical functions and mental faculties. What used to be an implicit claim to the right to health care is gradually becoming a claim to the right to health itself. What is more, people are not concerned with scientists' logical and methodological scruples; in France, quacks are consulted as often, if not more often, than M.D.s. And what we call medicine continues and develops in the middle ground between these two extreme attitudes.

Medicine's Successes

There has been much talk of "alternative" medicine, which as far as I know has not effectively contributed to combating a single identifiable disease. Yet what is pejoratively called "orthodox" medicine has been able to eliminate quite a number of once painful problems. Communicable disease is no longer a major factor in the death rate; some say this is due to progress in general hygiene and vaccinations, not in clinical medicine. This fails to take into account that, from Jenner to Salk, vaccines have been discovered through procedures typical of clinical medicine (fortunately, we did not have to wait until immunological science solved these problems).

Antibiotics have nearly wiped out tuberculosis; where it still occurs, they are saving millions of lives. It is significant that antibiotics were shown to be effective long before we understood how they work, a typical development in "orthodox" medicine that everyone seems to denounce today. Furthermore, although arthritis is still considered incurable, it is now rare to see it cripple people the way it did Raoul Dufy, who was forced to stop painting. More and more often cancer and leukemia patients see their lives prolonged by some years; in many cases where the life expectancy was once no more than a few months we wonder if it is not justifiable to say they are cured. Cardiac patients are brought back for additional comfortable years of life, while only a short time ago heart attacks were invariably fatal because of the immediate complications. Anticoagulants save lives every day, although the biological details of coagulation are still only imperfectly understood. Patients who a few years ago would have died within a matter of months from kidney failure are now kept alive with hemodialysis or transplants. Every day surgeons save patients who would have died given the same set of circumstances fifteen years ago. The list of all the progress medicine has made with "real" diseases—serious cases involving an imminent risk of death—would be endless. Thus it comes as no surprise that the demand for medical services is increasing, and that some people grow impatient or indignant when they learn that a doctor is not all-powerful.

I find it altogether remarkable that most of medicine's successes are arrived at through the empirical method, although, as we shall see, that does not imply an absence of methodology. Every existing science has been preceded by technical activity in the field, successive attempts at problem-solving, the exploration of a hitherto unknown world. It is clear that the empirical approach, besides being the only real option physicians have, will continue to produce advances. I will cite only one example, drawing on very recent and as yet very limited developments in the treatment of impotence. Since psychotherapy has had little if any success in treating the disorder, and drugs to cure impotence have not yet been discovered, surgeons decided to test penile implants. The first-generation prostheses were made of rigid plastic; the second generation are inflatable. Already there are men who have resumed satisfying sexual relations thanks to implants. This surgical procedure is still in its early stages and is still far from adaptable to all cases or successful every time, but it is nonetheless a superb example of intellectual daring, surgical engineering and the will to stretch the limits of what is possible. Medicine is not simply an attempt to understand how the human body works. It is also concerned with the human brain's challenge to the status quo. This is linked to the current widespread refusal to accept the decrees of fate or doctors' admissions of helplessness, a trend that both honors and alarms us as physicians.

Basic Sciences

In the medical school curriculum, those sciences not directly applied at the patient's bedside are called fundamental sciences: physiology, the various branches of biology, pharmacology and so on. Hence the temptation to which not only many basic scientists but also many clinicians yield: considering the physician's work as the application of the scientists' findings. A major mistake. Historically these disciplines arose from medical activity in the field, the persistent pursuit of the art of healing, in an attempt to answer some of the questions occurring to physicians in the course of their work. Little by little they became independent disciplines, and doctors continued to provide them with their raw material, as could easily be demonstrated by the example of immunology, a science that grew out of the practice of vaccination. In the intervening years, the clinical experience of physicians involved in treating cancer or transplanting organs has done more for "basic" immunology than immunology has contributed to the practice of medicine.

It is time this misapprehension was laid to rest. We should

grant clinical medicine its epistemological independence and its capacity to move on its own as it gambles against nature.

Exploring Experimental Models

Many researchers think the only difficulty they have to overcome is finding the experimental model of a disease. They can then use laboratory animals to solve the various problems in biological and medical science it poses and finally tell the doctor what it is he has to do.

Here again we could point out that the overwhelming majority of recent advances in medicine have been made without the existence of any corresponding experimental models. But that would not be enough. We must first demonstrate that every model is necessarily flawed and, more specifically, that no model can account for a disease's extraordinary heterogeneity in human beings, given the extreme genetic variation they display. Research either opts for simplification, working with one pure strain (the common practice in constructing an experimental model) and thus avoiding the situation that occurs in human medicine; or else, when possible, the disease is introduced into genetically dissimilar animals, resulting in so much complexity that it is no longer possible to deduce general rules.

The inherent flaws in experimental models are of little consequence in the study of disorders caused by such foreign agents as germs or toxic wastes. However, chronic or prolonged diseases involving complex mechanisms varying from one individual to the next do not readily lend themselves to the construction of an experimental model. Throughout the world, there are experts in the art of curing certain cancers artificially induced in purebred mice. Unfortunately, the results of the experiments cannot be extrapolated to human beings because physicians can observe cancer only when it has already succeeded in penetrating the body's defense system, thanks to a special set of circumstances governing the genetic potential of both normal and cancerous cells. The cancer cells have far more highly developed defense mechanisms than laboratory cancers do. The physician observing and treating cancer has to identify the ways in which the cells are able to survive and develop, then ask the research scientists how to go about studying countermeasures. In other words, in at least some instances, only clinicians are in a position to ask the right questions, since they are the only ones studying the real disease. Sometimes they must even come up with a likely solution and test it on their patients, as we have had to do with plasma exchanges in cancer patients.

The relationship of clinical to "pure" research is a fascinating subject, but is not the issue here. It must be admitted that pure research has its own irreplaceable methodology and applications. The problem is that medicine by its very nature not only operates in the realm of the uncertain but also has its own specific problem-solving technique, which has no equivalent in biological science.

Medicine as the Science of Troubleshooting

A "pure" scientist does not like the idea that a toothache can be treated by extraction, or gangrene by amputation, yet for more than a thousand years these procedures brought great relief to sufferers and saved lives. They were accepted and encouraged, and those who knew when to prescribe them and how to perform them skillfully were honored as the greatest of men, in keeping with the service they rendered. Ambroise Paré, fully conscious of how crude his art was, wrote: *"Je le pansai, Dieu le guérit."* (I tended him, God cured him.) But our collective memory is grateful to him.

Giving anti-inflammatory drugs for chronic arthritis, the accepted practice today, is no more "scientific" than prescribing aspirin for a migraine. Treating cancer with drugs that kill proliferating cells—almost as many healthy ones as diseased ones—may seem absurd. The only way to progress in these circumstances is to do everything possible to preserve the healthy cells, concentrating fire on the sick ones. Engineering tactics rather than scientific discoveries make it possible to turn these slow gains to the patient's advantage.

What can we gather from these examples? That unlike "pure" biology, medicine seeks to palliate, find acceptable compromises, ways of buying time. It seeks to prolong life rather than cure a disease once and for all. Perhaps the term "art of healing" is too ambitious and we should substitute "art of helping." The only true cure would mean eliminating death. Medicine proposes to hold death off as long as possible and is not terribly fussy about how it is done. Medicine accepts the idea of bypassing a blocked artery, even though it is a kind of surgical plumbing job. By the same token, if a tooth hurts too much, the medical cure is to pull it out.

Medicine is the science of troubleshooting breakdowns in the human body. No one expects the emergency repairs to work forever, or even for the body to work perfectly or exactly as before. But it must work fairly well and for a reasonable length of time. A diabetic cannot hope that his pancreas will be restored to its original condition, so he accepts taking medication every day of his life, waiting for transplants to become available. An amputee prefers wearing a prosthesis to not being able to walk. A cancer patient will undergo an operation, even a disfiguring one, if it removes the malignancy. And we are grateful to all those who do their utmost to find solutions—however inelegant, illogical or imperfect they may be at times—to the problem of staying alive and well.

What connects all this to the problem of decision-making under uncertainty is the fact that while a doctor is a repairman

—nothing more, but nothing less—there is no manual for what he is repairing. And the human body is a fantastically complex mechanism, far more complex than any conceivable physical system, even all nonintelligent biological systems. Moreover, the doctor is subjected to extreme constraints on his activity. He cannot take the body apart to find out what is wrong with it; he must make sure its vital functions are maintained while he is at work on it; and he must have the consent of the "machine." On the other hand he is allowed to take calculated risks (amidst the uncertainty) and sacrifice certain less important bodily functions to the essential ones when it is inevitable. A lucky doctor is one skilled at guesswork, since identical situations, to which a ready-made formula could be applied, are rare.

A famous and deserving Nobel Prize winner, Sir Peter Medawar, severely criticized the above thesis, which I outlined in an earlier work. Through the press, he let me know that there was no such thing as a pure scientist and that I had bad manners. I do not know why he felt threatened. But I do know something about attacks on physicians who try, as I have, to upgrade the scientific status of clinical medicine. Many researchers let it be known that they think they have nothing to learn from clinicians, and many clinicians agree with them. Even those who admit that applied research is possible and "profitable"—clinicians included—see it as limited to certain aspects of medicine and dependent on the same methodology that is used in laboratory work. Advances having to do with the best available decision-making techniques, for example—necessarily made in connection with cases that are not homogeneous and cannot be compared (since they resulted in different decisions)—are considered anecdotal, not scientific. It all comes down to a question of definition. Now is the time to open the debate.

CHAPTER IV

Research Medicine and Individualized Medicine

I *Clinical Research*

Many physicians believe they cannot contribute to the advancement of medicine, its body of knowledge or its power. They are wrongly convinced they are merely applying the formulas research has perfected. As evidence to the contrary, three goals have been defined for France's teaching hospitals: caring for the sick, teaching, and research.

Past advances in medicine were essentially the result of work on human subjects with the help of a methodology that, granted, was vague, hesitant and sometimes even dubious. Especially in the past few decades, it has become clear that the new means of treatment developed by biological research or chance observation or daring extrapolation can be directly proven only with sick people. It has become clear that experimentation with animals is a requirement in determining factors such as the maximum tolerable doses of certain medications, in discovering their potential undesirable effects and long-term side effects. Current legislation quite rightly provides for very complete biological studies of every new drug in various animal species and various situations (gestation, for example) before clinical experts are allowed to administer it to human beings.

It has also become clear that in addition to studying the effect various clinical procedures had upon the patient, the pathological process should be studied as well. This meant raising the huge problem of creating experimental models for human diseases. Thousands of researchers are working on either creating or identifying animal counterparts to human diseases. Their aim is to determine the development, the spread or remission, the various causes of these diseases, their sensitivity to pharmacological or surgical measures, and so on.

Today the experimental branch of medicine (founded single-handedly by the great Claude Bernard, or so it seems) is a major one, absolutely indispensable to the art of healing. In any number of areas it has shown itself to be particularly useful. It allows us to do testing much more precise and reliable than can be done with human subjects, since it varies only one parameter at a time in an otherwise stable context and is identical in all the subjects tested. That is the absolute condition for acquiring data that can be reproduced and generalized, for scientific knowledge.

Furthermore, experimental medicine theoretically eliminates any dangerous experimentation with human subjects. It is supposed to answer any question creative minds might ask without exposing human beings to undue risk. For these reasons, many experimental scientists consider the medical corps as no more than the drive shaft of experimental biology and pathology. They see doctors as the end of the process, following rather than initiating orders. And many doctors, as I have said, agree with them, believing that research with human beings is too difficult and dangerous. Within the last few years, however, an entire methodology of clinical research has developed on its own, and not by accident.

Today there are still problems for which animal experimentation offers no answers. Some diseases have no known equivalent in animals. In other cases the available models allow for no more than a crude approach to the reality of the disease. In still other cases the same disease, with a known cause, develops very differently in animals of different species and responds very differently to a single treatment. The result is that we have no idea whether a human being will have the same reaction as a rat, a mouse, or a chimpanzee did. Moreover, as I have already mentioned, the best models are still the simplified ones, fairly close but not identical to the human disease, not reproducing all its variations and the way it adapts in individuals, with all their differences.

We must therefore either resolve not to advance in these areas for the time being, or else find ways to eliminate or minimize the risk so that tests can be run with human subjects, providing us with new data and new ways of helping people. The latter choice would mean there is a need for clinical research, and that it should be filled.

A great number of research teams have made the choice and are successfully working in this new area of medicine. Often these teams include both clinicians and researchers, or their members may conduct both experimental and clinical studies. The specialists involved realize that this is untrodden ground, that the temptation to adopt debatable or even inadmissible attitudes is all too strong. Much discussion has ensued, with officials from various governments participating. Their goal is formulating a rigorous and unassailable methodology.

Methods and Applications of Clinical Research

Clinical research is not the subject of this book, but it seems indispensable to outline its methods and goals, if only to define by contrast the territory reserved for individualized medicine.

Curiously enough, to date very little has been written about the nature of clinical research, and the rare efforts to codify it contain considerable gaps. It is not anyone's fault; the problems involved are not connected to government regulations—except those ruling out certain practices hazardous to patients' safety and freedom.

Nevertheless, during the past few years important advances have been made in arriving at methodologies liable to meet with the agreement of the various groups and government authorities concerned. Precautions have been taken to guarantee that patients will not suffer from the treatments or procedures they undergo. As for clinical testing, it is used only on patients whose condition cannot be made worse by the treatment; at most, it will be less effective than conventional treatments. Moreover, the tests provide for very early detection of lessening of effectiveness, thus preventing any injurious loss of time. Finally, various procedures allow for built-in control groups so that statistical analysis can provide a clear answer to the question under examination (for example, "Is Treatment B demonstrably better than Treatment A? In what percentage of cases, and for what groups?").

These precautions show the direction clinical research is taking. Limiting myself to the therapeutic aspect, I will cite three examples of its applications, illustrating just how irreplaceable it is.

The first example deals with establishing the area of effectiveness of a new anti-cancer drug. Meticulous experimental studies have shown that a new product, or rather one chemically derived from an existing product, has been effective against a group of transplanted or induced tumors in animals. This means there is a good chance it will work against tumors in human beings, but it is currently impossible to predict the extent of its effectiveness on various malignancies appearing in different organs, not to mention its effectiveness compared with that of drugs already available. Other research studies have defined the drug's dosage within acceptable limits of toxicity. This dosage should allow us to explore its effectiveness against a wide range of cancers, in the hope of finding a use for it in treating malignancies of the lung, digestive tract or bone. At first we treat only patients whom available, potentially active drugs have not helped so that they will not be deprived of possible beneficial effects. As a result, the new drug may not do as well as expected in the test, since all drugs administered after an initial treatment has failed prove less effective. We would rather run this risk, however, than deprive the patient of a well-founded chance of getting better.

If our first clinical study establishes that the product in question is active, according to quantitative criteria I will not go into, in at least 20 percent of patients, we will not hesitate to begin using it as a first treatment in the hope that 40 percent or more of patients will respond to it. After that, more complex tests will determine in what sequence it is best to use the new product, which by now will have become part of the therapeutic arsenal. Should it be used first, second, or in conjunction with an already established treatment?

Another question among the hundreds that might be asked now occurs to the clinical investigator who has tested the new drug. This leads to my second example. Should the optimum dose of the drug be administered all at once or over a period of three, four, or five days? The question should be more specific still. If there is something to be gained from spacing the dosage, is it more important for one type of tumor than another, or more important for slowly growing tumors than for fast-growing ones?

The third example is linked to the same set of questions. What *is* the optimum dose? Are there any genetic differences that could account for the fact that the drug is effective in only 40 percent of patients for whom it is prescribed? Could it be that some patients inactivate it rapidly, giving the drug no time to work? Isn't the real problem to find the optimum dosage for *each* patient? I am happy to bring up this problem, because it has just been very elegantly solved by a team of Marseilles pharmacologists working with an anti-cancer drug that has long been available and active, but which should now prove much more effective thanks to their work.

These examples illustrate, I hope, the specificity of clinical, and more particularly, therapeutic research. There are not at present any studies with laboratory animals that provide answers to the problems I raised. It is also easy to see how random clinical observation, or even an accumulation of observations not corresponding to a precise and predetermined design, could not provide the answers. A clinician settling for this kind of observation without following the methodological and statistical rules of a therapeutic study would expose himself to working from unfounded impressions, being swayed by his own illusions (what statisticians call biases) and thereby making mistakes—well intentioned, yes, but no less wrong for that.

Thus we can see that clinical and therapeutic research is an attempt to reduce uncertainty. In the field of human medicine, it represents a means of acquiring controllable data before getting on with business. It requires the study of large numbers of patients in order to overcome the obstacle of the heterogeneity of the groups treated and result in valid conclusions.

It is therefore tempting—and every clinical researcher I know all over the world has experienced this temptation—to think that if experimental research is not medicine's ultimate tool, then clinical research must be. In this light it appears as the loftiest, most scientifically profitable form of medical practice, and individualized medicine by contrast seems to be only the pure and simple mechanical application of the results of clinical research.

I do not sanction this widespread idea. Now that I have pointed out the absolute necessity for clinical research—which takes up a good deal of my own practice—I must describe its apparently constitutional weaknesses and show why the advances in research in no way lighten the physician's awesome task: deciding under uncertainty for each individual case.

Weaknesses and Limitations of Clinical Research

We have seen that to ensure an appropriate comparability of groups studied, especially in regard to therapeutic response, the researcher must treat a large number of patients in the hope of attenuating or compensating for biological differences of an unknown nature that can exist from one patient to the next. The danger here is that the study will give a clear picture of the average response to the treatment, but no idea of individual reactions. It is good to know that Treatment A is better than Treatment B because it is effective in 40 percent of lung-cancer patients instead of 25 percent. But the decision-maker remains unsatisfied. He knows that more often than not the statistics are the result of a cooperative study by several groups, and for inexplicable (or explicable) reasons, the results, which varied greatly from one group to the next, were simply averaged. This problem, linked to the essentially statistical aspect of a clinical study's results, is far from being solved (except in the case of a medication that proves to be active in 90 percent of the subjects tested).

There is another limitation to therapeutic studies that merits discussion. Protocols for clinical trials always note the fact that the researcher is basically acting in the interest of the patient under treatment, and that the treatment can therefore be changed at any time. What the guidelines are trying to measure, however, may be how long a product is active in treating a chronic disease. They must therefore set up criteria for failure, which the participants in the study agree to acknowledge and follow, and without which it would be impossible to calculate how long the drug did remain active. It can and does often happen, however, that to eliminate any ambiguity and ensure reasonable comparability from one group to the next, the criteria for failure require such strong proof of progression that it is quite obviously a waste of time.

In a study on mathematical models for tumor growth, my coworkers and I have shown that failure of a treatment could be dated from the exact week when continuous regression stopped, and that following international guidelines could lead to the loss of two or three months, sometimes more, before the treatment was changed. Yet it is easy to understand how clinicians engaged in cooperative research want to go along with the game and send the research center directing the study observations it will deem usable. Not to mention the countries where secretaries, research nurses and equipment are partly paid for with money brought in by the production of such observations.

This can result in serious conflict between the task of reducing the uncertain to the certain (the goal of clinical investigation) and making the best decision for each individual case (the physician's natural vocation). And this is not the only conflict. To be effective, a therapeutic study must deal with only a minimum of questions, ideally one at a time; for instance, whether Treatment A or Treatment B is better. In other words, all the patients participating in the study will receive either Treatment A or Treatment B exclusively until there is demonstrable failure or recovery. Only in this way can the biostatistician overseeing the study reach valid, publishable conclusions on which the international medical community can draw.

A few years ago I had a disagreement with the representatives of a certain international cooperative group about a situation I thought a good illustration of the excessive and unacceptable inflexibility of these therapeutic guidelines. The disease was cancer, but that is not important here. Suffice it to say experience led me to suggest treating it with a sequence of chemotherapy, surgery, radiotherapy and more chemotherapy.

Simply comparing this therapeutic sequence to the conventional chemotherapy treatment most groups adopted would be fraught with enough difficulties, the biostatisticians thought. When I specified that nothing would happen on a fixed schedule, that the intensity, type and timing of each of these treatments would depend on the patient's response to the preceding one and his or her tolerance for it, the reaction was outrage. How could any conclusions be drawn from a therapeutic program with such heterogeneity? How could we even propose such a study, comparing patients receiving different doses of radiotherapy, different lengths of chemotherapy treatment, and even, in the second sequence, different chemotherapy, depending on how they had responded to the first round? How could there be a single group including patients whose surgical history was very different due to the extent of the remaining malignancy and the various techniques of excision used?

All this was considered unreasonable, and the project was turned down. What struck me at the time, and still strikes me, is that my failure in fact represented the triumph of biostatistical thinking over the medical concept of service and established the principle of rejection of any strategy based on individualized decision. This type of study had too many parameters and too many different circumstances for a statistical analysis to arrive at significant conclusions. There was no choice but to rule it out and limit studies to what is statistically provable. I pleaded that I had probably gotten better results than I would have with the conventional procedure, that it was the statistician's job to invent new evaluative tools and not the physician's job to use only those methods today's statisticians are able to evaluate. My plea was in vain.

Is the only solution to work in obscurity, treating patients according to our better judgment, but in such a way that our peers cannot or will not hear about what we are doing? My coworkers and I have not found an answer to this question, but in searching for one I have come across two potential solutions, which I will offer here as food for thought.

The Feynman Solution

Richard Feynman, a renowned statistician and Nobel Prize winner, came to Paris at the invitation of a mutual friend and spent an entire day listening to my differences with the statistical community. He was not particularly familiar with the medical aspects of what I described to him, but he was very quick to catch on. At the end of the day he could only advise me: "For every new case in which you want to try using a sequential strategy of your own devising, you could bring together a panel of experts, ask them to examine the patient and give a prognosis based on the use of a conventional treatment. If your own treatment does better than the best the experts predicted for the conventional treatment, it will then be worthy of consideration."

I do not know what professional biostatisticians will think of the idea, or if the editorial board of a medical journal would allow such data. At any rate, in my work environment it is not feasible to convene a panel of experts to look at every new case, so I have not been able to test Dr. Feynman's suggestion. But I offer it to all those who might have occasion to apply it.

The Calman Solution

Kenneth Calman is head of the medical cancer unit in Glasgow. He and I have discussed the problems of clinical research many times. Here is his solution: A written record should be kept of the sequential strategies that might be applicable to each type of disease, specifying when, how, and based on what data the decision to change treatment would be made. Then every time there was a new case in which one of these strategies might be used, we would choose at random either the sequential treatment we consider best or the best available conventional treatment. A statistical analysis would subsequently be possible, comparing breast-cancer cases treated with each method, for example, then ovarian cancer, and so on.

This is an attractive, intelligent proposal, but it would be difficult to apply. It would require a great deal of time, and also that 50 percent of patients be treated with what we do not consider the best method of treatment. There have been times when I have told patients: "I have absolutely no idea whether Treatment A or Treatment B would be better for you in the long run. And no one else knows, either. Do you have any objections to a random choice?" Even so, I can hardly imagine myself saying: "I think that Treatment A is better than Treatment B, but we're going to choose at random because not everyone agrees with me."

There is quite obviously a serious possibility that my judgment is faulty and that these personalized strategies, involving sequential decisions according to different indications, may not turn out to be any better than the single-method, monolithic strategies being used in most of the international clinical studies now under way. If I am the one proposing the changes, it falls to me to prove I am right. But I have not as yet been able to settle on a procedure that might eventually allow me to do so.

In any case, perhaps this discussion has at least made clear that no physician can consider himself relieved of his responsibilities as a decision-maker, even if he is participating in cooperative clinical research, even if he hopes to make a personal contribution to the advancement of medical science in a form acceptable to the scientific community.

A few concrete examples are probably in order at this point. I beg indulgence for their inevitably technical character. I will choose them from an area with which I am familiar.

CHAPTER V

Examples of Decision-Making Under Uncertainty in the Treatment of Cancer

TREATING CANCER is a prime example of decision-making under uncertainty. My work as an oncologist was in fact what led me to seek out logical models. For at least a decade, a succession of drugs and techniques has superseded conventional methods of treatment. Not that we know everything—far from it—about the spectrum of activity of these new weapons, their effectiveness, their side effects in the middle and long term and the best way to combine them with one another or with already existing methods of treatment. To complicate matters further, the individualized characteristics of both patient and disease are largely responsible for a malignancy's development and the response to various treatments. Finally, it takes a long time before we can say for certain that a cancer has been cured (fortunately this is happening more and more often nowadays). It is easy to understand, then, why there are differences of opinion and a high degree of uncertainty about choosing the best therapeutic course.

Yet sick people come to us every day. In our field, delaying a decision is not an option. Every cancer specialist can tell when the prognosis is good, statistically speaking, provided a well-defined treatment is followed. In the majority of cancer cases, however, there is nothing to lose, because left unchecked the disease would spread rapidly and fatally. A decision has to be made, and made under uncertainty. Even if the decision is to do nothing, the physician is just as responsible as if he had decided on a treatment.

With examples chosen from my specialty, I now hope to illustrate what I have already said about the dimensions of uncertainty. We will be dealing with situations that are not cut and dried, since either no controlled clinical study on them has been done or none has been conclusive. If different specialists were to suggest what might be done in these situations, they would have differing opinions. This may seem surprising, but in fact it is the general rule when working under uncertainty. No one would expect a group of generals to give the same solution to a problem of strategy. Obviously, not every strategy is a winning one. We can therefore expect several of them to succeed, with variable losses, even though they are not identical. Likewise, several others will fail. Medicine is no different, and part of my discussion is intended to examine whether it is possible to improve medical decision-making.

This chapter is not a neutral listing of different options. My goal is to evoke the concrete situations in which my coworkers and I try to rationalize our therapeutic choices, working against uncertainty. I have indicated what we base our decisions on and why we prefer them to other common courses of treatment. We will be open to criticism if there are flagrant errors in our logic. We hope this is precisely what will happen so that we will know how and what we are doing wrong in certain instances. In other words, my proposal is that the various strategies should be discussed before the battles are waged. It would mean not only pooling more of our gray matter but also seeing how we could do things better, how we could weed out potentially harmful preconceptions, logical stumbling blocks, inertia and fashions in medicine.

Early Detection: Deciding on Localized Treatment

It is generally agreed that a newly detected tumor should be removed if it is operable. There is still some discussion about certain tumors of the breast, head or neck, for which radiotherapy may offer other options. But even in cases where there is theoretical agreement, concrete courses of action differ, sometimes inexplicably so.

Surgery for lung cancer is a good example, to my mind. In some cases the only possible surgery is pneumonectomy, or the complete removal of the lung, either for technical reasons or because of the extent of the tumor. In others, the reverse is true, and only a lobectomy—the removal of one of the pulmonary lobes—can be performed, since removing the entire lung of a patient with a long history of smoking, for instance, would further endanger his respiratory capacity. In many cases, however, either type of operation could be performed, and the surgeon must choose between them. In the overwhelming majority of cases, the lobectomy, the more conservative operation, is chosen. The justification for this involves a true error of logic which many thoracic surgeons commit: They look at the survival statistics for the two operations, find them very similar and infer that for equal results the less serious and less incapacitating surgery is preferable.

They are forgetting, however, that patients selected for lobectomies have traditionally had the least developed cases of cancer, while pneumonectomy is used in more extensive, thus more serious cases. The question is this: Wouldn't the success rate be even higher if patients now undergoing lobectomies were given pneumonectomies? Everything points toward it, since we know pneumonectomy is the best way to eliminate cancerous ganglions that may be present in the mediastinum. Localized relapses, a very serious occurrence, are more likely after a lobectomy than a pneumonectomy. Finally, like many other types of cancer, lung cancer is often multicentric. After a lobectomy, microscopic tumors may remain in another part of the lung, capable of subsequent growth and metastasis. Some surgeons see red when they learn their colleagues are not performing radical mastectomies, a practice so common that it is no longer challenged, and no one seems to remember there are alternatives.

Another problem of logic in thoracic surgery concerns very extensive surgery in cases where the pericardium, chest wall or atrium is involved. Very thoroughly documented studies in the United States have shown that the prognosis for major operations in these cases is bad. Surgery may save 50 to 80 percent of patients with small tumors, but only 10 percent of those requiring extensive surgery. Thus the trend is to prescribe surgery only when it is considered useful and to steer toward a palliative program of treatment, radiotherapy or chemotherapy, in other cases.

French medicine generally does not take the same position, and fortunately so; otherwise what would happen to the 10 percent of curable cases not receiving the surgery they need? It might be argued that this means only one out of ten patients operated on will be saved and the other nine will undergo needless, painful, not to mention costly surgery. There is a solution, however: various tests determine which patients with extensive malignancies have a real chance of being helped by surgery. And we know, at least theoretically, that the prognosis is best when certain features of the immunological system are still functioning, or when the tumor's growth rate is slow. So if there are doctors who feel they should refuse to perform ten operations in order to save one patient, we can screen patients for them and make their operations more profitable, medically speaking, without sacrificing the 10 percent of patients who will benefit from surgery. It is simply a question of stating the problem clearly, keeping all the givens in mind, discussing objectives and optimizing measures step by step. If the new approach needs to be tested, the methodology of clinical research is available. What we should try to avoid are generalizations based on righteous arguments with a semblance of statistical support; their proponents do not even realize they are beside the point.

Extensive abdominal surgery is another good example. Every day, all over the world, patients are operated on for cancer of the abdominal cavity. Surgeons have very different attitudes toward similar cases of the disease in the same stage of development. This would be all to the good if the variations were the result of decisions based on an analysis of individual characteristics. That is not, however, always the case. Here again we must single out extreme situations, when there is no choice but to follow the course dictated by the state of affairs. In the early stages, the ganglions in the immediate area of the malignancy are removed along with it. When a malignancy is so fully developed that removing it would entail unacceptably radical surgery or very high-risk surgery with only temporary positive effects, the cancer is left untouched.

There are, however, intermediate cases in which surgical daring can make all the difference. It does not depend on any particular technical skill, only on the operating surgeon's confidence in what may be gained from extensive surgery.

For instance, my hospital was sent a patient from Eastern Europe for medical treatment after the removal of an intestinal cancer. The operation was recent. It had not affected two metastases in the liver, which were isolated and operable. Why? If the surgeons had thought that metastasis in the liver, no matter how isolated, wiped out the patient's chances of survival, why did they send him hundreds of miles to be hospitalized, to undergo a treatment they did not believe in? If they thought the postoperative treatment had some chance of succeeding, why hadn't they helped to make it more effective by removing the two metastases when they had the chance?

My coworkers and I, among others, have observed that when ovarian cancer has spread to the abdominal region before it is detected, subsequent chemotherapy is much more effective if the surgical "shrinkage" of the malignancy was complete. Some surgeons, however, still send us patients whose exploratory surgery was not followed up with the painstaking cutting away of malignancy that can change everything. Why? There are even surgeons who use different tactics from one ovarian cancer patient to the next; there is no way of knowing what they will decide in a given case. Do they themselves know? What are their secret criteria for decision making?

Controversy is also raging in the crucial area of choosing an initial treatment for breast cancer. The options are many, and I have no intention of using this discussion to explain my own choices. The only problem I will raise is that of coherence in individual treatment.

Initially, there were no alternatives. The standard treatment was a radical mastectomy: removal of the breast, pectoral muscles and armpit nodes. This surgical procedure was devised a century ago for malignancies detected at a much more advanced stage than they are today. Later, with the advent of radiation therapy, the use of x-ray treatments before or after surgery was proposed. More recently, surgeons have tried to leave as much of the breast intact as possible. The following strategies have evolved: removing the malignancy but leaving the healthy portion of the breast ("lumpectomy"), with radiation therapy for the remaining tissue and the ganglions; radiation therapy only for small malignancies; and implanting radioactive material in the tumor to give a high concentration of localized radiation, followed by generalized radiation of the affected area. Lately a new dimension has been added to the debate: postoperative chemotherapy, which some physicians recommend when the armpit nodes are affected (and finding out that they are means removing them).

There is thus a broad range of choices. Each has its supporters. They exchange rationales and statistics, naturally; better yet, they specify the factors entering into their decisions: size of tumor, breast size, presence or absence of palpable ganglions. No matter how heated the arguments get, the reasoning is worth it if it leads to the development of a logical tree of decisions, offering the best compromise between safety and aesthetic considerations in each case, or else providing a choice between maximum safety and a compromise, and so on. My own position in the debate has remained firmly based on logical argument and biological fact, plus a precedence for safety over aesthetics. I am quite ready to change my thinking and the treatment I offer, however, if new evidence convinces me that certain choices I have hitherto ruled out are in fact acceptable ones.

The existence of aberrant strategies is another problem altogether. Why does one doctor suddenly depart from logic and prescribe a strange sequence of treatment? Why does a surgeon who usually performs "total" nonradical mastectomies occasionally opt for more limited surgery, with unconventional doses of radiation therapy afterward? In certain cases of bilateral tumors appearing several years apart, why will the same surgeon, or the same radio-surgical team, adopt a radically different strategy in each case when there is no biological or anatomic difference at all? Why do some physicians completely reject certain methods of treatment without ever examining them as options in cases where they might have something to offer? In medical problem-solving, which is essentially finding ways to make the best possible decisions under uncertainty, categorically rejecting certain therapies is as inadmissible as deviations from the norm (which ideally has been defined in a logical way).

Clinical studies clearly have a role to play in the attempt to reduce uncertainty in this domain, as my friend Bernard Fisher of Pittsburgh, director of the National Surgical Adjuvant Breast Project,* agrees. One day, thanks to his efforts and those of the surgeons participating in his study, we will know if the partial removal of the breast (breast "segmentectomy") is as safe a treatment for cancer as removing the whole breast. We will know the odds no matter where the tumor is situated, what size it is, the state of the accompanying ganglions, and whether or not postoperative radiotherapy or chemotherapy is used. This will require ten years of study, however. Bernard Fisher contends it could be completed much more quickly if *all* breast-cancer patients participated.

But for many reasons, good and bad, that will never be. And so despite the fact we will be immensely grateful to Dr. Fisher ten years from now, until then our decisions will have to be made on a basis that, if not strictly personal, we consider rational rather than scientific. How we should improve our reasoning is the immediate question for those of us not in Dr. Fisher's group of researchers.

The Problem of Systematic Postoperative Chemotherapy

A great many national or international clinical studies now under way are exploring the potential benefits in the treatment of cancer of a variety of combinations of chemotherapy administered systematically over a long period. The question is

*A national study of postsurgical adjuvant treatment for breast cancer, one of the projects the National Cancer Institute funds.

whether patients, or certain subgroups, see a postponement or elimination of possible recurrence with these treatments. At the same time, the ratio of advantages to disadvantages is being worked out, determining whether the potential benefits are outweighed by unpleasant side effects or even toxicity or complications.

Curiously enough, the mere fact that these studies have been undertaken is enough to infuriate doctors who have made up their minds (on what grounds we do not know) that postoperative chemotherapy will never constitute a valid recourse. If a study with negative results is published, their loud rejoicing is heard; when a positive study comes out, they dispute it, questioning the authors' scientific honesty or declaring that the results are too preliminary, or claiming the "risk" of publishing results before ten years of study is too great, and so on. Attitudes like this are nothing new in medicine, and indeed in all other scientific disciplines as well. They have to do with a certain kind of pathological behavior that it is unfortunate to see in fields where we are working to reduce uncertainty for the common good.

Nonetheless, a very thorny problem remains. What about the vast majority of patients, those not participating in the controlled studies I have been referring to? Should we wait three years, or ten, or take a calculated risk with them? In France, the doctor is the sole judge of this. In many cases where an American physician would not take the risk of proposing a treatment "before the results are published" (for fear that failure or complications with the treatment might result in a malpractice suit), a European doctor is still fortunate enough to be able to follow his own conscience in deciding whether an available treatment might improve the prognosis in a specific case—and then prescribe it.

No scientific evidence will ever be drawn from a mass of cases that cannot be compared to one another, that are treated by different doctors and without reference to a control group of untreated cases. But that is not the problem at hand. The formulation of unambiguous answers to questions as important as this is indispensable; it can be done only through rigorous studies flawless in their methodology. But until we have the answers in hand, must we dispense with any supplementary treatment in all individual cases? Do we have to agree that the prognosis for a certain situation will remain unchanged while we spend ten years waiting for a study to be completed? Or can, *must* a practitioner decide to try something more for each person who comes to him for help? At this point in our experimental and clinical knowledge of the results of chemotherapy and immunotherapy, I can give as an example my own group's position, expressing nothing but choices based on our preferences and our personal evaluations of the available data.

It has been shown that certain cases have a high probability of being cured by surgical means alone. We then find it inappropriate to take risks or prescribe a treatment that might eventually prove harmful; we do not want to interfere with the delicate equilibrium that allowed the body's defense system to surround the tumor and keep it from spreading. In such situations we tend to rule out chemotherapy unless indicated by further developments. But other treatments may be useful: hormone therapy, vitamin A derivatives, immunostimulants, as indicated by the situation and by test results. Here our first concern is not to interfere with the natural healing process.

At the opposite end of the spectrum, malignancy in certain organs has not been shown to respond to any type of chemotherapy, even an anecdotal case. By this I mean that in cases of identical inoperable tumors, no chemotherapy to date has brought about an observable shrinkage which might encourage us to believe that elsewhere, in cases of microscopic tumors left behind by surgery, it might prove effective. Here again, we would not use chemotherapy, except in controlled therapeutic studies. The drain on the body's resources is not worth the hope of possible improvement. And here again we would have no objection to prescribing a less aggressive course of treatment, such as immunotherapy, provided the effects on the immunological system have been tested.

As always, between these two extremes lie a vast number of cases in which chemotherapy has proved effective in treating a certain percentage of established tumors, which were advanced enough at the time of surgery to cause concern about the probability of postoperative recurrence. This is where the decision-maker must act. Nothing has been published about them, often nothing is due to be published for years, allowing us to believe that rigorous studies will prove largely positive. But we cannot be sure whether the chemotherapy we are using will entail a percentage of long-term complications, or whether the percentage will be negligible (as has proved true for radiation therapy). Here we are inclined to propose a prolonged postoperative chemotherapy, estimating that the patient has more to gain than to lose from it. We also make the treatment proportionate to the seriousness of the case. In other words, lighter doses than those for inoperable tumors are used, and every possible precaution is taken. And of course we are ready to stop the treatment if it appears that the patient's tolerance is too low.

I must say that I would not hesitate to decide on this kind of treatment for myself. It has also received a vote of confidence from the many doctors who refer members of their family to us and from the patients to whom I explain the different courses of treatment available to them. I readily concede, however, that it is not universally accepted.

A problem with this approach concerns patients who learn (often by accident) that the operation they underwent a year earlier was for cancer and then come to us after the fact to ask if systematic postoperative treatment is necessary. If x-rays and biological testing uncover the first signs of recurrence, which is not yet producing any symptoms, that is evidence enough of metastasis. Then there is no question about beginning treatment. But if the tests show no such evidence, and the cancer was a type with a good prognosis to begin with, the patient need only be closely watched. If it is a type for which chemotherapy would have been suggested at the outset, I propose the treatment on principle, despite the time that has elapsed and the absence of any symptoms. What would I do if the operation had taken place two, three or four years earlier? Probably nothing, but it would be a special case, an individual decision. (I should note in passing that this brings up another type of problem. By what means, and how often, should we check up on a cancer patient who is not receiving treatment? Physicians' answers to this question are many and varied.)

Lifesaving Situations

Today's cancer specialists—radiation therapists as well as medical oncologists—are consulted much more often in last-ditch situations involving metastasis and recurrence than they are when the disease has first been detected. The typical outline, slightly less common today than it once was, is this: An operation is performed by a nonspecialist surgeon, or a specialist in the diseased organ; then there is perhaps radiation therapy, followed by firm opposition to any generalized treatment or even any consultation with a cancer specialist; then, if there is a recurrence, comes dismay. More often than not, the family or the patient seeks the help of a cancer specialist because the original physician is convinced nothing more can be done.

Occasionally we see a variant on these positions which is absolutely unjustifiable in logical terms, whether it is taken by a general practitioner, a surgeon or an accredited cancer specialist: "Let's not do anything now, let's wait to see if there's metastasis." Chemotherapy, however, is effective roughly in inverse proportion to the number of cells in a tumor, and if metastasis is bound to show up later, some microscopic evidence of it must already be present.

All this notwithstanding, oncologists gladly deal with the most advanced cases. The success rate with them is of course relatively low, and this fact is used to justify not sending newly detected (and much more easily curable) cases to cancer specialists. Yet oncologists generally, if not always, accept the challenge. What I call last-ditch or lifesaving situations, many others would call hopeless or terminal. This aspect of oncology, which is so difficult and so large a part of our work, no doubt poses the greatest number of problems in decision-making, with a wide range of results from one strategy to the next. I will try below to give examples, indicating in the process how great the need is for a general debate on these problems in decision-making.

Surgery for metastases is becoming increasingly common. We have long known that an isolated pulmonary metastasis of a cancer originating in some other organ can be surgically removed, sometimes adding several years to the patient's life expectancy. Doctors and surgeons have slowly reached agreement on how best to identify the patients who would benefit. There must be a single metastasis, appearing several years after the primary tumor was removed, and it must have a slow growth rate.

Is it possible to formulate an effective strategy even when all these conditions are not met? In the United States, I met a healthy boy who two years earlier had had twenty-seven pulmonary metastases removed: a seemingly desperate attempt that was successful. In France we have not been quite that audacious, but we do recommend excision in cases where it has not conventionally been an alternative. The choice of excision is based on these criteria: a small number of metastases, three or four, taking more than a hundred days to double spontaneously (meaning it would take them from five to eight years to increase from a diameter of one centimeter to ten centimeters) or else clearly regressing under chemotherapy, which leads us to believe that chemotherapy during the postoperative period would be likely to eradicate the still microscopic metastases associated with the ones removed surgically. This treatment has met with very encouraging success, but also failure (new metastases appearing six months to a year after surgery). Yet it still seems to me the best choice we have to offer in a situation where doing nothing means no hope at all.

Many factors, obviously, may influence our decision-making. We would be very hesitant to recommend this treatment for an elderly patient, or for a younger person with cardiovascular irregularities that would make the operation itself risky and very aggressive in therapeutic terms. We may be able to improve on this strategy. Practically every day thousands of cancerous cells travel through the lungs when there is a tumor elsewhere in the body. If several years after initial treatment the number of metastases is very limited, then we presume that for various reasons the host of other putative metastases has been destroyed or blocked. Is there any way we can help the lungs with their cleaning process? Perhaps there is, with anticoagulants, with immunostimulants, especially when they are administered in aerosol form. Years of study will be necessary before we can establish what there is to gain from these techniques. What can they do for a patient now? We tend to combine them with postoperative chemotherapy if there is no medical reason not to. Looking for ways to optimize decision-making under uncertainty implies adhering to a logical framework—within the limits of our present knowledge—and continually striving for improvement and innovation, making the most of every new discovery or technique.

Can we extrapolate the above to dealing with metastases in

other organs? It would be rather bold to do so, especially since the lungs can be minutely explored with x-rays, while organs like the liver or brain require the use of scanners, a new and not readily available technique, though not yet as refined as x-rays for the lungs. Nevertheless, if the conditions listed above are met, if the metastases are in addition located in operable areas, some surgeons do not find it unreasonable to suggest operating, while making it clear how uncertain the results are. Today patients are surviving for appreciable amounts of time because medical-surgical teams have offered and carried out such treatment. A decision like this, made under uncertainty and with one's back to the wall, is hardly even a decision. It is simply a case of determining if the treatment seems reasonable in a given situation. If the answer is yes, there is no way to justify hesitating. Discussing the ultimate results of our actions, however, will mean having to spend a great deal of time defining the word reasonable.

Should we give up or go on? We have to ask ourselves this painful question much more often than we would like. How can we tell when it is time to call a halt to treatment? We are torn between wanting to take every case as far as possible—not to prolong life expectancy by a few weeks, but rather to keep open the possibility, however slim, of real and lasting improvement—and sparing the patient a treatment heavy in side effects if it is unnecessary. Even before the factors in the decision have been weighed, the doctor is subjected to sometimes contradictory pressures. Some family members would rather "get it over with" and others demand that everything be tried, even in a terminal situation. What about the patient? It is very rare to hear a patient ask that attempts to save him be stopped. Quite to the contrary, he most often listens closely to his doctors, asks his nurses why treatment has been suspended. He does not try to talk to the doctors about it but looks for signs that medical measures have been abandoned, which would mean that those entrusted with caring for him have lost all hope. We are aware of this as we make our final decision.

Sometimes it is easy. All the available methods of treatment have failed, or else the patient's body, in particular the bone marrow where new blood cells are formed, can no longer tolerate the medication required. The medical team's job then becomes alleviating pain and giving as much comfort as possible in other ways. I have had conversations with exhausted but lucid patients in that very situation; I number them among the most excruciating moments in my life.

Even more remarkable, however, is the fact that in all good conscience medicine sometimes abandons patients who could still be treated. What right have we to give up on a human life? One argument is that it is what the patient wants, that our insistent treatment should not interfere. In fact it is the other way around. The cases I will now describe, a few examples out of hundreds of similar ones, involve patients who came to us of their own accord after they had been given up on by the physicians who had been treating them.

One woman came saying, "I have hepatic metastasis of a primary breast cancer. I had a mastectomy a few years ago. The doctor I've gone to since my surgery told me: 'You have about three months to live. There's nothing more I can do.' What do you think?"

I thought I could hardly believe my ears, especially since the hospital she mentioned was rather conservative about telling patients the truth. Her husband, as deeply affected as she was, confirmed everything she said. The specialist seems to have made two decisions simultaneously: to tell the patient what he considered the inevitable prognosis as bluntly as possible, and to reject any attempt at treatment even though the patient had not been following a therapeutic program since her operation. My coworkers and I began treating her several months ago.

The metastases have shown considerable regression. Our patient comes in every two weeks, under her own steam. She jokes with us. She is waiting to see what happens, and we are waiting with her. Some identical cases fail in the middle term. Others are entirely stabilized after four years, as medical teams all over the world are well aware; we are not the only staff with this kind of program.

Age is another factor in decision-making. A seventy-year-old widower was diagnosed as having inoperable cancer of the stomach. He was given a prescription for painkillers and sent home. The diagnosis was not spelled out for him, but he guessed it. He thought things over for a few weeks and decided to try his luck. He had lived a very full life, full of sound and fury during the Resistance. His wife had been beheaded by the Germans. Once his mind was made up, could his doctors possibly question it? They did, and the more so since they were convinced nothing could be done for him. My coworkers and I advised radiation treatment (beyond any doubt an unorthodox method for gastric cancer), then oral chemotherapy treatments. He lived for two more years without missing a single day of treatment.

We are now treating two very young men with inoperable lung cancer, both smokers and, obviously, turned away by the physicians they first consulted. The first man was told his diagnosis in detail, the conclusion being that nothing could be done, that radiation might have a palliative effect later, when the pain began. He thought this over for a few weeks, then revolted against it and came to ask us if there was really nothing to be done. I think that even if I had been convinced there was no hope for him, I would still have set up a therapeutic program to make him feel that someone was caring for him, that he did not have to face his crablike inner sickness alone and unaided. It so happens, however, that our long, well-documented, published experience convinces us that attempting treatment is legitimate, that spectacular regressions do occur, lasting six months to two years and longer, with sequences of treatment we are now perfecting. The young man's treatment is under way.

It has already proved successful with one of his fellow patients, who traveled five hundred miles to us by ambulance, hovering near death, because his wife refused to give up on him. Today he is back on his feet, at home. His lung is clean. How long will it last? We do not know; no one does.

Considering the success we have had with our program of treatment, we cannot help questioning the decision to do nothing which is usually made in similar situations, in France and elsewhere.

Often the physician must decide whether or not to preserve a bodily function. A young woman had a fibrosarcoma removed from her forearm, followed by radiation therapy. She was under the care of specialists. A local recurrence went unnoticed for three months, until it could not be missed. There was a radical change in the specialists' attitude. Emergency amputation at the elbow was recommended. Beside herself, the young woman decided to consult several different medical teams. We offered her the following plan, which she accepted: interarterial chemotherapy, through the arm, for ten days, to achieve a very large localized concentration of drugs in the spot where the malignancy had recurred; simultaneous hyperthermia (therapy involving heat to affected areas); dissection and removal of the tumor, which would mean partial loss of function in one finger; then prolonged chemotherapy in her hometown, under our supervision. Nearly a year after the operation, she is radiantly healthy, and her hand works almost perfectly. We cannot be sure that her cancer will not recur. If that were to happen, we would have to discuss amputation. But our experience has been that there is a good chance of completely controlling the disease, and she still has her arm.

What is more, a patient like this also runs the risk of metastasis, particularly in the lung, which amputation would not affect. Chemotherapy gives her added protection.

Here is another, almost identical case. A former policeman was stricken with sarcoma of the shoulder blade. Disarticulation of the shoulder, a total removal of the shoulder and blade, was recommended, an extraordinarily disfiguring operation, but reasonable under the circumstances. He refused the surgery and was sent away. If I had thought the operation was the only course open to him, I would have told him so; I often confirm other physicians' opinions (yes, there *are* times when doctors agree). But this man had just retired, was otherwise in good health, and thorough testing revealed no detectable metastasis. My decision was to put off the recommended operation, try a combined program of radiotherapy and chemotherapy, and continue chemotherapy for two years. The sequence was completed nearly four years ago. My ex-patient and I get together once a year to celebrate his good health. The most interesting aspect of the case is that other doctors at the medical center he originally went to would certainly have suggested similar treatment. It is a hospital with an international reputation for radiation therapy with bone cancer. But the day our patient was advised, the decision-maker in charge had other ideas. Or perhaps some personal problem . . .

Determining priorities is an important issue. Should everything be sacrificed in the hope of a possible recovery, or should a bodily function be preserved even when it is not absolutely safe to do so? Where do we begin in a difficult situation? Sometimes it is best to work first toward general well-being and comfort; sometimes radiation must be done before anything else. In other cases chemotherapy must be considered an emergency treatment and undertaken at once. In still others we must ask ourselves whether a life-threatening cerebral metastasis must be attacked, or whether it is more reasonable to treat it only if we are certain we can at least stabilize the other quickly developing tumors in the body.

Determining the best therapeutic sequences is often difficult. There are cases where we know a recurrence in irradiated tissue will not respond to chemotherapy because the tissue has become fibrous and poorly irrigated, and medication does not penetrate it. Then, counter to all our acquired habits and the reigning inertia, we must make sure that an operation is performed, followed by chemotherapy, then radiation therapy to clean up the area. Sometimes it is the other way around, because a malignancy that can be cured by radiation therapy is a quickly growing one. Even if it is very extensive, even if radiotherapy will mean a long delay, for various reasons, in the generalized chemotherapy that is still necessary, we must begin with radiation treatments, and if need be ask the therapist to devise a shorter-than-usual sequence.

When are we justified in combining all these measures at once, if we are unable to decide between them, and still protect the bone marrow as much as possible, since its continued functioning is vital to prolonged treatment? The answer depends on the patient—his age, earlier treatment, physical condition. Today we can tell how the problem should be set up, but it seems almost impossible to give all the answers before the fact—in other words, to foresee every variation nature can produce. Yet this is exactly where our efforts toward progress are leading.

Let me add that any projection extending over a fair amount of time of course runs a great risk of being proved false by an unforeseen factor: failure, complications, toxicity, unexpected improvement. . . . Almost every day I get a letter along these lines: "One of my parents is too weak to be transported to your hospital. This is his/her condition. Could you please send an outline of the treatment you would suggest for me to give to our doctor here?" That is like asking a bridge player to explain how he will play without any knowledge of what his opponents' plays will be.

For these difficult cases, the patient's presence is required. As in many other medical specialties, in oncology some phases of the disease demand direct involvement in the game, a game that can last for years. In other phases, fortunately, the family doctor can handle most of the work with the help of a few phone calls and an occasional appointment with the oncologist. It is clear that the way hospitals work must be modified to meet the needs of modern medicine, but that is another story.

CHAPTER VI

A Phenomenological Survey of Medical Decision-Making

WE HAVE NOW taken a look at levels of uncertainty in the practice of clinical medicine and considered specific examples, taken from my own special field, of decision-making under uncertainty. At this point, before considering remedies to what is quite obviously an unsatisfactory situation, it may be useful to ask ourselves what really happens at the moment a decision is made: what factors are taken into account, under what conditions, and how lucidly.

I do not believe any attempt has yet been made to do this, and my own approach will necessarily be only a partial one. I must rely on my own recollections, which go back to the time when I did not make a conscious effort to think in terms of decision-making under uncertainty. My insights into what other doctors experience are only more or less exact. As I have said, I began to see the light after years of simply wondering what logic had governed the previous treatments of patients I saw in a critical state. At times I would not have treated them differently; medical oncology does involve losing many patients. Often, too, though I was convinced another treatment would have been more effective (much easier to say with hindsight), I could discern a coherent therapeutic position and a line of reasoning. What dumbfounded me, however, was that often I could not reconstruct a line of reasoning, penetrate a decision-maker's system of logic, pick out the inconsistencies or judgments based on incorrect gathering of data.

The sum of my thinking, the failed treatments I had to understand in retrospect, led me simultaneously to look into decision analysis—which I will discuss later—and the phenomenology of decision-making in the medical milieu. A series of sketches will best illustrate what I imagine, although I am well aware of the technique's limitations, its distortions and summary nature.

The Unknowing Decision-Maker

This is the most usual case, and the least offensive one. Here is a doctor who has earned an M.D. without ever having been told that decision-making is his prime function. Since he has always done his homework, he knows that such and such a case or situation implies such and such therapy, which he applies without further thought. He is little inclined toward abstract speculation, and his mind is not easily changed. If he experiences failure, he may decide to do something different the next time around. But his choice will be almost instinctive, with no real abstract formulation of the courses open to him. Something decides for him. Let's hope it works for the best, since this kind of doctor will never realize that in making a decision he is choosing one of a handful of possibilities, each of which in turn introduces new choices. He works more on reflex than reflection, relying on an intuitive combination of what he knows and remembers. He may also instinctively push aside cases requiring overly delicate choices, referring them to his colleagues. He works essentially in the realm of certainty, where he can prove very useful. As we shall see, the majority of character sketches below are also covered by this definition. It is the rare doctor who knows he is making a decision. Yet at least the unknowing decision-maker functions unselfconsciously and smoothly. Perhaps an encounter with doubt is all he needs to turn him into a true healer.

The Ignorant Decision-Maker

I tend to think this is a rare specimen, probably much rarer than some people think. To put it simply, someone who doesn't know an answer generally knows he doesn't know it, and does not make a decision. There have been a few flagrant exceptions, even among the teaching staffs in medical centers. For the most part, however, ignorance is not a very great threat in medicine, nor does it alter the decision-making process. Subtle flaws in knowledge, conscience or character are far more dangerous. This does not mean that our era does not have its own special problem with information. Knowledge grows and replaces itself so quickly that doctors must spend hours every week poring over medical journals, trying to sort out the crucial information. There is no solution in sight. It would be wrong not to give our patients the benefit of the very latest in medical care. What can we do to keep from getting six months behind? We subscribe to journals publishing summaries of articles, and read hundreds a week. We await the help of data processing and its obedient electronic memory banks.

A first step would be for doctors to lose their fear of admitting ignorance or difficulty with certain cases, and for patients not to conclude a doctor is not a good one if he does so. This two-sided misunderstanding, this communications gap, has been responsible for problems that are both regrettable and avoidable.

It is impossible for today's doctor to keep up with everything new in medicine. He must be allowed to confess his ignorance; it in no way interferes with the quality of care he gives, since patients can always be referred to physicians with more knowledge of their specific complaint. The only real problem is when a doctor has illusions about how much he knows, or thinks nothing has changed in the past five years. If he is persuasive, his patient may end up believing this too.

The Cautious Decision-Maker

Caution is almost always a virtue, especially for a doctor or surgeon. But as we have seen, certain situations require an evaluation of opposing risks. A minimum-risk strategy can always be devised, but not always applied; in some instances it would lead to a minimum-gain situation—in other words, failure. Could the cautious decision-maker be mainly concerned with his own peace of mind? As malpractice suits multiply, this is becoming an issue. We will all be tempted to stick with the tried and true, not to try to work surgical wonders but to remain within the limits of the possible, laying the blame on nature rather than therapy. It will obviously be up to the public to choose what kind of medicine it wants: an optimal medicine, with all the risk it involves, or a minimal medicine.

With this in mind, there are also genuinely cautious, overanxious doctors who would always advise against any bold step, even if it represented the patient's only chance. The family assents, waiting for a situation that can only get worse to go ahead and get worse. And who is to say they are not often right?

The Careless Decision-Maker

Here we are no longer talking about optimal medicine, but maximal medicine. There are far too many examples to choose from. The decision-maker takes every risk, ending up with complications and treating them with catastrophic results. He is not in control of the procedures he uses. Thus a friend of mine had his leg amputated at the thigh (but was not cured) after a clearly excessive and therefore inappropriate treatment. A few years ago, in his inaugural lecture as professor of thoracic surgery at the University of Paris, Dr. Mathey said something that still stays with me: "Unlike a bus driver, a surgeon risks only one life at a time, without risking his own in the process." This is equally true of any doctor. Hence the absolute necessity of keeping one's head, never forgetting what is at stake: the life of a human being. Our profession precludes athletics. A doctor can take all the needless risks he wants when mountain-climbing, but never when making a therapeutic decision. A surgeon dazzled by his own skill, daring and brilliance should stop operating. His job is not to show off, but to care for others. The same holds true for any doctor who might be feeling smug after a string of successes. As professionals, we must be entirely free of self-indulgence. Henry Miller said it somewhere in *Sexus* (I quote from memory): "It's very easy to be a good doctor. Just forget about yourself."

The Hurried Decision-Maker

It is easy to run into him in any hospital as he rushes from one case to the next. He is immensely weary. He wants our sympathy, wants help with the heavy cross he has to bear. His caseload is too big, he can't go on, he works impossibly long hours. Fortunately, however, the voice of an oracle speaks through him. Without pausing for breath he makes important decisions, decrees a grand strategy in the wink of an eye. He can charm, inspire confidence, even be content with his choices. But how often?

A friend of mine once took a relative to an appointment with this kind of doctor. Her description of it was revealing. "What an extraordinary man! He had only three minutes to spare. You could tell he was tired. But he still got up and examined my cousin. He wrote out a prescription without another word and then said goodbye to us. The nurse told us his whole day would be like that."

We should not conclude too hastily that the doctor in question was relying on instinct rather than reason. But I have never forgotten the story. The hurried decision-maker is a dangerous individual. Furthermore, sometimes he is not really pressed for time but is simply a "born hurrier." With this type of personality, he cannot take time to think. He likes being overburdened with work, or else he is afraid of what he might find out if he slowed down. Chronic haste can be a psychiatric disorder. Then why is the right to care for others, and make choices, handed out with an M.D. to less-than-well-balanced people? This is a difficult problem, one we have not addressed and perhaps never will. It would seem that to practice medicine a doctor should be sound in mind. But who would have the exorbitant privilege of determining whether or not his peers are sound in mind?

As for the decision-maker who really is in a hurry, who sees more than a reasonable number of patients, he should be made to slow down. Just as we no longer applaud the virtuoso surgeon (the kind who could remove a stomach in less than an hour), the virtuoso decision-maker should also disappear from the scene. Medicine is too important to be practiced by people who never have time. They are short not only on time but on good judgment as well. How can they allow themselves to form an opinion without listening to the concerned party, without making the effort to understand the patient, pinpoint his doubts and unformulated questions, gauge how committed he feels to a complex therapeutic program?

The Unpredictable Decision-Maker

He always has an opinion: that is for certain. But he changes it constantly with the circumstances. Once I asked my friend Bernard Fisher how he thought our colleagues made their decisions. He replied that in the overwhelming majority of instances, a therapeutic decision was arrived at in direct relation to what happened in the last similar case the doctor was familiar with. I am afraid he may be right, that for the majority of potential deciders nothing takes precedence over the emotional impact of the last case they have treated or seen again, no matter how different it was from the one at hand. If a therapy, however coherent, did not live up to the doctor's expectations, there is a strong probability he will not apply it in the next similar case.

This is like betting heads every time after tails turns up, and vice versa. It is a dangerous attitude because it shows a total lack of confidence in nature's workings and ultimately in all causality. Or in any case a lack of confidence in our ability to deal effectively with the causality which we perceive as chance. Uncertainty is not haphazard, and that is why we can use strategies against it and improve on them. Those who find it impossible to believe that our choices made under uncertainty can become rational should get out of the profession.

The Depressed Decision-Maker

He has lost faith. He is tired. He has invested a great deal, both intellectually and psychologically, in his self-image, and he has experienced a string of failures. Nothing holds interest for him any longer. Why should his patients have to fight? He calls a halt to therapy, the excuse being the patient's poor tolerance, for instance. When I reconstruct stories like these, the patient routinely tells me: "It's not that *I* couldn't take the treatment, my doctor couldn't." That is true, and it happens often. Does it mean the doctor basically lacks confidence in the medical profession? Or will he recover his enthusiasm in a few months? In any case, it is better for someone with medical problems not to consult a doctor going though a depression. The damage can prove irreversible.

A well-known surgeon operated on a woman with abdominal cancer. Exploration of the lesions showed the disease to be much more extensive than had first been thought. The surgeon, a friend of the patient, despaired of trying the large-scale excision he might have performed and closed the woman up, bursting into tears on the husband's shoulder afterwards. My coworkers and I later treated the woman, keeping her alive and active for more than four years. I believe we would have done even better under different circumstances.

A colleague phoned me about a patient we were both following. His lung cancer had entirely stabilized for eighteen months, thanks to monthly chemotherapy treatments that kept him in bed, exhausted, for forty-eight hours each time. "I can't take it anymore," the doctor in charge of the case told me. "I just dread his infusion sessions. Why should they have to go on?" Yet when I talked to the patient, he protested, begging that the sessions continue.

The Sadistic Decision-Maker

I think I have already given some examples of this type. He orders amputations for young patients when avoiding them could be a calculated risk. He removes the ovaries of young women operated on for breast cancer when no other factors in the case justify such a move. Or else he announces to the patient: "You have three months to live," or perhaps "Come back when the pain starts. We'll see if we can give you some relief. That's about all we can do."

His conscience is untroubled; he is doing his job, and like all sadists he would be amazed if you were to point out this character trait to him. He is perfectly unaware of it. In his private life he is no doubt a wonderful person, for he fully satisfies his sadistic impulses through his work. Once again, we touch on the problem of doctors' mental health.

The Temperamental Decision-Maker

He roars when someone asks him a question. He loses his temper if his patient tells him he wants a second opinion. He refuses to send records to other doctors. In short, he literally cannot bear to have his decisions challenged. His irascibility is not a good sign. If his decisions are well-founded, he has nothing to fear from a confrontation. In addition, he would lose nothing if a prospective patient were to decide not to work with him. On the contrary, patients are grateful when a doctor graciously engages in a discussion they may well feel their lives depend on.

But the temperamental decision-maker does not care what his patients go through. He institutes a reign of terror. How often, when it seemed time to send a letter to one of my colleagues summing up my opinion on a patient of his I had just seen, has the patient stopped me, saying, "You mustn't write to Dr. X. He doesn't know I've been to see you. He wouldn't take it at all well." I then wonder what a patient is going to do with an opinion no one will ever hear. I usually insist on writing anyway, sending the most natural letter I can, making excuses for the patient, inventing some relationship between us, a mutual acquaintance, so that the doctor will not be offended (it doesn't always work).

A longtime patient of mine was a very young woman with metastatic breast cancer. Her initial therapy had been quite strange. The doctor in charge had strongly advised her against coming to see me when the metastases appeared, telling her nothing more could be done. She lived four more years, leading an active life, and her metastases shrank to some degree. But when she eventually ran into the doctor in question at a dinner party in their small city, he bitterly reminded her of the prognosis he had given (which she reported to me during her first appointment). Unfortunately he proved right in the end. Her death must have been a great boost to his ego.

Here I would like to tell the present or future medical students among my readers that they will never be faulted for hesitating, for admitting their trouble with a difficult case or their inability to handle it, for requesting one or more outside opinions. We do not practice medicine to create or bolster a self-image, but to serve as best we can with all our shortcomings. The whole secret is to recognize the latter and not try to hide them. There may be patients who expect doctors to have presence, be articulate and quick to decide; that is their problem. There may be doctors who are trying to prove something to themselves through their work; they should get out of medicine and seek power somewhere else.

The Inconsistent Decision-Maker

This is perhaps the most dangerous type. He is missing a few links in terms of logic, or else he functions in a non-Aristotelian system, not respecting the law of contradictions. Curiously, though, this holds true only for his work; in everyday life he is perfectly pragmatic. But as far as medicine goes he is not what decision theorists term "consistent." He will construct a strategy aimed exclusively at controlling a situation with only a 5 percent chance of occurring, and will neglect to take other elementary precautions in the case. According to his mood, he will react in a radically different way to two identical situations. He is totally unpredictable. Reconstituting his decision-making process by studying a patient's case history can be a real puzzle. He decides on a therapy that is not imperative, halts it for unfathomable reasons, then goes back to it later with only the slightest modification. I continually ask my interns to note the reasons for our own changes in position on our patients' records. Whether or not they are valid, they remain on file so that we can understand them ourselves when we review the case, if need be, to pinpoint our errors. Nothing is more disconcerting than a vain attempt to piece together the reason behind a change of course. But the inconsistent decision-maker is not disconcerted; it is not in him to be. In one instance he will prescribe a low-dosage chemotherapy sequence in a serious situation. This is dangerous because the cells build up resistance; soon what was initially the correct dosage becomes too low. The next time he will order intensive chemotherapy for a situation with a good prognosis. In one case he recommends that a treatment usually carried on for eighteen months be cut off at six; in another he adds a drug that has already proved ineffective.

The Falsely Systematic Thinker

Here we have yet another species. He certainly does have consistency, but with no reference to reality. He has formulated a few ideas which he applies no matter what the situation. They may have to do with the way surgery should be performed, the nature of a medical treatment, the composition of an imaginary subgroup of patients for whom he does one thing rather than another. It is no use reasoning with him, or presenting counterarguments. He pays no attention, goes on as before, perhaps attracting followers for a certain period. This is what happened to a well-known French anatomist-pathologist (may he rest in peace) who decreed that pulmonary adenocarcinomas in the lung had to have migrated from another organ and could not possibly originate in the lung. As a result, for years patients with this disease were subjected to an avalanche of costly and useless examinations looking for their "primitive cancer." They were the only patients in Europe or the whole world for whom therapy was delayed or denied, since our sage held that their lung cancer could be nothing but metastasis. And the fact the 90 percent of the time all the tests came back negative did nothing to shake the certainty of the movement's leader or his disciples.

In this chapter I have limited myself to a few quick descriptions. We have seen that the traits likely to have a negative influence on the decision-making process are many and varied. There are purely factual parameters, related to a lack of information, negligence in data gathering or poor organization. There are others having to do with intellect. The inability to think logically is a serious failing in a doctor, particularly as he is working with the latest developments in medicine. It is clearly a problem for patients if their doctors suffer from irrationality (just as politicians or military men may). Another threat comes from fanatics whose logic does not refer to reality, and who are among the most dangerous.

But as we have also seen, in many cases the factor with a negative influence on the decision-making process is tied to the physician's character, his personal neurosis. This is a crucial observation, although it is only common sense. It is not at all certain that achievement tests or rigorous medical-school standards would give us mentally sounder men and women more likely to be in control of their performance. There is at least the same percentage of neurotics among doctors as among plumbers or business executives. And it is true that doctors do have an inherent power, the same way aerospace engineers have power over airplane design and electricians over home-building. We would simply like to be certain that this power rests in good hands. Now that decision-making has become a large part of medicine, this is a problem that we will not be able to ignore and that should be taken into account in all planning for the selection of future doctors.

Finally, while I have discussed the demands we must make in our logic, I have not mentioned moral considerations, one of the prime, the most authentic concerns of a good decision-maker. We will take a longer look at this question after a survey of decision analysis.

CHAPTER VII

A Medical Reading of Decision Theory

As I have already said, I first looked into decision theory for practical reasons, not simply to improve my mind. The bibliography lists the works I found accessible; I hope I have understood them correctly. I learned a great deal from them. Here I will attempt to communicate only the points that apply directly to the practice of medicine. So far no decision theorist has written a book about medicine; it would be of great interest to both mathematicians and physicians.

Putting medicine aside—and it is not mentioned in any of the works I consulted—decision theory makes very encouraging reading. It is good to see how the human mind is determined to advance, how undaunted it is by the unknown. Are there areas of uncertainty? Fine. Let's work on them. First let's catalogue them, differentiate between them, see if there are identifiable species in the vast sea of uncertainty. Then for each category let us see how we can make the consequences of our actions less uncertain. Let's see if we can at least partially foresee them, if they can be assigned a coefficient of probability. Let's find ways to evaluate the results of our choices (the "minimax regret"* criterion is one I find particularly thought-provoking). Finally, let us introduce strategies that will reduce the proportion of chance in these outcomes. If I have understood correctly, all this is already under way. Today's mathematicians are carrying on the work of Pascal, Bernouilli, Borel, Von Neumann. Economists, military strategists, top managers in business use the tools of decision analysis, or at least those available today. It seems to me that this attempt not merely to speculate but to orient our actions in a still essentially unknown universe corresponds exactly to the situation in certain sectors of medicine and offers concepts with direct applications to the practice of medicine.

Objectives, Goals, Finalities

Decision theory carefully distinguishes between objectives, goals and finalities. Beyond any doubt this is where we should begin a discussion touching on the very heart of medical activity. We are concerned with therapeutic decisions under uncertainty; no valid decisions can be reached until these concepts have been analyzed.

An objective is the quantified expression of a goal. For example, we could define our *goal* as curing breast cancer. Our *objective* would then be curing 40 to 60 percent of the cases of one kind of breast cancer. The concept of *finality,* or ultimate end, is so crucial that I have devoted an entire chapter to it. Several books would be better. I am addressing it here in order to stress the way in which evaluating goals and choosing objectives hinge upon it. We know that in an identical case different strategies will be developed by one doctor who considers that a human life has to be fought for as long as there is awareness, and another physician who thinks that

*A minimax strategy seeks to minimize the maximum possible loss.

some diagnoses automatically imply nonintervention, "therapeutic truce" or treatment exclusively aimed at bringing comfort. It might seem that there are no general rules, only specific cases. This would mean every doctor is an objective, rational being, and that all doctors share the same set of finalities, have the same conception of the best way to serve. This is very far from the case. Unfortunately, it is rare enough for doctors even to think deeply about the problem of finality; it can take years of sometimes painful inner searching to enrich this thinking. Medical school, it is true, does nothing to prepare physicians for it. Each doctor must do it for himself, guided only by personal beliefs or preconceptions. Furthermore, only those with a taste for general ideas will do this thinking at all.

The problem is discussed at more length in the next chapter. But we can already see that a clear conscience about finalities informs, or should inform, the entire debate on decision-making. As Geoffroy d'Aumale put it: "The formulation of finality is an organization's philosophical (perhaps even political) expression of itself. Unless the finality appears permanent, there is profound internal disorder." The same author remarks that there are hierarchies of finality and that they should not be tampered with. He cites the finality of the Defense Department, which leaves off where a superior finality begins (constitutional principle, for instance). Some groups (such as economists) might be strongly tempted to think that the finality they represent takes precedence over medicine's. Whatever the case, at this point in our examination of finalities we can see that defining them borders on the determination of goals. For example, a physician's view of finalities can determine whether or not he would operate for lung cancer.

If my personal conception does not rule out treating a patient with widespread and not completely curable cancer, I will set myself the goal of finding the best palliative treatment possible. This may eventually entail telling the patient in some detail about the different steps to be taken—for instance, surgery to reduce the size of a tumor, followed up with long-term maintenance therapy with drugs, the added precaution of radiation therapy at a certain point, and so forth. If, on the other hand, my innermost conscience told me that "gaining" a year or two would not be worth the unpleasant effects of the treatment or the trauma revealing the diagnosis would cause, then my goal would be to mislead the patient radically about his situation and not use any specific treatment. Or I might reveal the diagnosis if I believed I could not choose to withhold such vital information, but advise against any specific treatment, indicating I thought the game was not worth the candle. There are even more delicate aspects to consider. If I choose to tell the patient the diagnosis but explain the reasons for my pessimism, what will my attitude be if I then have to begin therapy anyway because the patient demands it? All too often I have seen patients referred to me by their own doctors leave our center with detailed therapeutic instructions, then be given only part of the prescribed dosage, or have their treatment delayed or needlessly interrupted without consulting us, simply because the patient's physician, in all good faith, "didn't believe in it."

In terms of goals, there is one instance in which the conflict can be even more delicate for certain doctors. Where the current state of our knowledge allows us to expect that a fairly long palliation is possible, certain doctors will still decide against therapy. But what about areas where treatment has already been shown to "cure" 15 to 20 percent of those receiving it, while the rest are simply given a "prolongation"? Should we treat a hundred patients to cure only fifteen or twenty, or should we keep on abstaining from treatment because fifteen or twenty out of a hundred is not "enough" to justify the effort, cost, side effects and so on? Or even, after enthusiastically embarking on this course, with the feeling that saving fifteen or twenty patients makes it worthwhile, can we then go back on our decision after the thirtieth straight failure and give up because we did not see the successes first? Perhaps this illustrates the complexity of determining goals in decision-making under uncertainty and in areas so fraught with responsibility.

Determining objectives is not a particularly easy task either. Let me once again use a definition of Geoffroy d'Aumale's: in decision theory, an objective is "the quantified expression of a goal."* It is readily apparent that this definition applies directly to industry or the military. The same is not true for medicine, where quantification is emphatically not always possible and where sometimes conflicting objectives have no quantitative resolution. As an example of the first instance, many doctors and patients are advancing the idea of "quality of life." In concrete terms, this means that surviving longer, or even being cured, would be only as valid as the quality of the life gained as a result. There is no denying this noble concern. But how can "quality" be quantified? And who is to decide what is acceptable in terms of quality? Doctors, well people or sick people? Today some attempts are being made to evaluate comfort or discomfort by having patients fill out questionnaires. Data gathered in this way can only be subjective, obviously, and more closely linked to the patients' survival instincts than a neutral measurement of their relative comfort. Furthermore, patients can only be questioned about what they have already experienced, meaning that often treatment must be undertaken first and evaluated later in terms of comfort.

With that in mind, there are instances in which a consensus is easily reached. I can formulate, and propose to the patient,

*Another definition of "objective" in decision theory is "the outcome that is desired by the decision-maker" [translator's note].

the objective of a cure requiring some type of amputation, and get a clear-cut answer from the patient and his or her family. On the other hand, I cannot conceive of a "cure" that would involve the loss of speech or awareness. I do not know how a young woman will react if the operation we propose, the only one practicable under the circumstances, involves a colostomy she will have to deal with for the rest of her life. Should I try to influence her decision?

Finally, there are critical situations which may produce conflicting objectives having more to do with tactics than strategy. The goal is to attempt the cure of a fast-growing tumor through aggressive therapy. Should we bear down to make sure the tumor does not "get away," or should we let up so the side effects will be eliminated and the patient will be able to eat and sleep better?

This distinction between the interwoven concepts of finality, goals and objectives has led us to dissect the intellectual activity underlying the medical act and perceive a basic level of priorities in therapeutic decision-making. There is much more to be said on the subject. We shall see that a reading of decision theory will bring up many additional questions.

Decisions Under Risk

Although an individual therapeutic decision is very rarely made in a situation of extreme uncertainty, it is valid at least to mention the criteria decision analysis has developed for evaluating uncertainty (that is, when the outcomes of the various possible courses of action cannot be ranked in any order of relative probability).

- The *optimistic criterion* uses the strategy with the greatest proportion of favorable outcomes.
- The *maximin utility principle* calculates the worst possible outcome (minimum gain) for each possible course of action.

The least bad course of action (the one with the maximum minimum gain) is considered best. This is also known as the "pessimistic criterion."

• The *Laplace criterion* favors the strategy with the highest average conditional outcome.

• The *minimax regret criterion* calculates the maximum regret (difference between the payoff obtained and what the best course of action would have yielded) for each course of action and opts for the one with the minimum maximum regret.

The risks involved in a course of action are usually assigned a numerical probability. More specifically, the various events that would result from this course of action are expressed in terms of probability. The conditional gains each of these events might represent can be averaged out to express what can be hoped for from this course of action. A Bayesian analysis indicates the best course of action, corresponding to the highest average factor of hope. For each of the courses of action compared in this way, then, the greatest risk, which corresponds to the least desirable outcome, must be evaluated. The maximum risk a situation can bear without deteriorating must then be defined, and Bayes's theorem used to eliminate those courses of action that might carry too great a risk.

At this point we should define an unjustifiable risk in medical terms, yet there can be no one general definition. It is linked in each case to a patient's earlier condition, the risk we run if no therapeutic action is taken (state of the illness, whether or not the vital organs are threatened, and if so, when), the risk engendered by the various therapies, the patient's preference, and so on. Certain situations may be judged lost causes, excepting the hypothesis of getting the maximum result from a strategy also involving maximum risk.

If the situation is life-threatening unless an operation with an 80 percent mortality rate in the context is performed immediately, it is probable that all surgeons consulted in the case would agree to try the operation, and that all patients and/or relatives would find the risk acceptable. But how are we to reach a decision if the maximum risk means a loss of bodily function, causing serious and irreversible problems? We should at least know about the probability of this maximum risk. There is no proof that Bayes's criterion—using the strategy corresponding to the highest average hope—would be of any use here, if it leads to an unacceptable alternative.

Even before the decision stage is reached, we see how indispensable it is to have evaluated risk. Astonishingly, some physicians seem to make instant decisions. Perhaps they are born decision-makers, capable of determining courses of action, evaluating and comparing their respective risks, almost by reflex. But what if this is not the case? What if an uncalculated risk occurs in a situation in which the elimination of all but minimum risk is imperative? And once again we cannot blame today's doctors for not using methods they have never been informed about. It is high time to alert them to the existence of decision analysis, acquaint them with the mechanics of decision-making we are almost entirely oblivious of even though we use them constantly.

And then again—here we come back to the problem of finality—who is evaluating the risk? What kind of person is he? What is his background? What concessions is he ready to make? What will his outlook be? Does it include humility? This calls for further discussion. It will not be easy to come up with a profile for the ideal decision-maker.

Objective Probabilities

We have seen that evaluating a course of action not only means forecasting the various outcomes, but also assigning them a probability, the sum of which is equal to 1. In decision-making under uncertainty we do encounter cases in which probabilities can be assigned on the basis of objective information. This is true for events with a distribution shown in a mathematical law such as Gauss's law or Poisson's law. The probability of certain events can easily be calculated; it is then possible to compare courses of action in terms of the various criteria described above. It can also happen that the decider is unable to assess possible outcomes in this way but does have data on their frequency from published studies. We now know, for example, the range of toxicity for specific dosage of every active drug, and whether or not cumulative toxicity is a threat. We also have a relatively precise idea of how often a given treatment ends in failure and even in which organs recurrence is most likely to appear first. If there are various drugs available, each with different effects upon different organs, we can use this knowledge in formulating strategies likely to reduce the rate of failure. This is what has happened in therapy for acute juvenile leukemias in which certain "sanctuaries"—organs where leukemia cells can develop unaffected by the drugs commonly used to fight them—are reached through special therapeutic procedures.

It goes without saying that the medical decision-maker's knowledge of these "historical" frequencies comes not from specialized literature but from his own experience. In other words, his experience must first be translated into usable data. This brings up an important practical problem. As long as doctors in medical centers have such limited access to secretarial skills and computer time, there is a great risk that their irreplaceable experience will be lost to science.

A related problem is equally important, if less obvious: it is very easy to deceive oneself about one's own experience, most often out of sheer optimism. How many of us are tempted to say that a given therapeutic procedure we were the first to adapt or apply, or which corresponds to our own theory of the cause of a particular phenomenon, has a 50 percent yield of improvement or cure, while the true figure is nearer 20 percent? The reverse is true for dyed-in-the-wool skeptics, who see all human effort as doomed; they report only their failures. A doctor's experience is rarely clear-cut. I readily agree that the art of medicine has its basis in experience, and it is one field where deciders get better results as they grow older. But it is not a linear relationship, since memory colors and transforms real experience. It is imperative to preserve experience in the form of data accessible to all and available to correct our mistaken impressions or recollections. My co-workers and I decided to use private gifts to our center to fund our archives. We have acquired a computer and are building a data bank with the help of the entire medical staff (and a consulting computer specialist). We have done this in part so that we will be always aware of the confines of our experience. Making an estimate or an error can introduce uncertainty where there could be certainty; no one in our profession can afford to do this.

Subjective Probabilities

In some circumstances it is virtually impossible to estimate objective probabilities (based on observed relative frequencies). It might be said that no two medical cases are alike, considering physiological differences at the outset, whether the disease is evolving rapidly or slowly, and the variable effects of medication. If on top of everything else a combination of treatments is being used, the therapeutic and toxic effects do not interact identically. Then no model, experiential or otherwise, can estimate the relative probability of the various possible outcomes.

In this sort of situation it might well be possible to act without an assessment of probabilities, as in a situation of extreme uncertainty, and adopt a live-and-learn attitude, so to speak. But we quite rightly expect more of a doctor: he should at least clarify the situation, explore and elucidate his reasoning if he cannot depend on facts. This is what he usually does. Decision theorists have repeatedly addressed this problem, which still seems to give rise to heated controversy.

I do not plan to discuss the concepts of deterministic versus stochastic dominance* in relation to the decision-maker's "rationality" (see Batteau and Marciano in the Bibliography), since they involve more mathematics than I care to include. Let me say only that there are probabilities dependent upon information that cannot be expressed mathematically: experience, expertise, memory and so forth, and we can help the decision-maker assign a subjective probability to one or more outcomes by offering him reference decisions which will at least give him a rational basis. Leonard Savage (Saint-Sernin discusses his work in detail) formulated an axiom of subjective probability, stating that it measures a rational individual's belief in the truth of a particular proposition. It is not my purpose here to describe the debate between the "subjectivists" and "objectivists" nor to explain how others have reconciled the two approaches. Once again, see Saint-Sernin. His book showed me that observing the rules of compatibility of beliefs means we can combine relative frequency and the degree of likelihood of various events in one mathematical operation, and how this can lead to more successful strategies.

I would, however, like to reiterate an idea of his which seems to me to be essential: the decision-maker must have a code of consistency. In other words, the probabilities he assigns to given outcomes are connected and governed by laws, which

*"As opposed to a *deterministic* decision rule, which keeps one on the 'best' road, a *stochastic* decision rule recognizes that there is some value to exploring alternate routes occasionally to see whether in some cases one of them might be better than the 'best' road" [Bursztajn et al., *Medical Choices, Medical Chances,* Delacorte Press (New York, 1981), p. 159].

means that some beliefs are incompatible, inconsistent, contradictory. It is admissible for two deciders to have a different evaluation of the same situation occurring in nature. But it is not admissible for a single decision-maker to be incoherent, at least when others' lives are at stake. Rigorous logic thus appears to be the sine qua non for determining the probability of uncertain events. I do not know of any tests that would measure a medical decision-maker's consistency; I hope decision theorists will develop some.

The ins and outs of decision theory have more to do with everyday medical practice than one might think, at least when we are dealing with illnesses whose outcome is uncertain. We often see inconsistent therapy, founded on fantasy rather than reality. This is the case with the treatments offered by quacks or "alternative medicine" fanatics. They are based on no specific observation or any law inferred from experience. They are deduced from an imaginary representation of the world, of supposed "connections" between human physiology and a nonorganic, spiritual or other universe. There is no longer any question of assigning justifiable subjective probabilities to possible outcomes of a therapeutic act: we are dealing with dogma.

On the other hand, however, how often do we run across doctors who, when faced with a logically justifiable therapeutic proposition—justifiable precisely because the probabilities of uncertain outcomes are correctly evaluated—simply and curtly say, "What proof do you have that this will work?" Asking for proof when working under uncertainty is a much more widespread attitude than one would think, and a particularly harmful one in that it stifles innovation. Admittedly, it is often possible, even indispensable, to test a therapy experimentally before applying it in a clinical situation. But that is not always the case. Medicine is a day-to-day affair: confronting pain, deteriorating health, the need to find an answer here and now. It is not acceptable, I repeat, for a decision-maker to be inconsistent. Nor is it acceptable for a trained decider to be prevented from imagining and implementing remedies to an otherwise hopeless situation.

Combinations of Certainty and Uncertainty, and Decision Trees

Mathematicians have fully understood that outside of a few very simple situations in which time does not alter the parameters, even certainty presents the decision-maker with a series of successive choices depending on whether certain natural occurrences (which may have known causes) enter into the decision-making process. As a result, there are hierarchies of experience (for example, more experienced doctors will make different decisions); judgment and conjecture are an art. Saint-Sernin cites Napoleon on the "divine" component of military strategy and the "inspiration" Plato attributed to Themistocles.

When nature is our opponent, certainty and uncertainty are most often combined in variable proportions. If we calculate the possible consequences of an action, we arrive at several possibilities, some representing the direct consequences of that action, others the combination of those consequences with occurrences beyond our control. From here we estimate the possible outcomes of further actions. The diagram of our analysis is what theorists call a decision tree.

Each "chance node" or "choice node" (or fork or point) is evaluated in terms of probability, objective if we have the necessary data, or subjective if we do not. We shall also see that each has to be assigned a relative value or "utility." To the extent that we can predict the various possibilities stemming from each "move," this gives us a diagram of the whole game, revealing the best tactics. A chess problem might be solved in this way. Saint-Sernin compares making decision trees and extending them to choices involving a combination of certainty and uncertainty to "Pascal's analysis of games of chance through endgames."

An underlying assumption is that making a decision tree requires not only assigning a probability to each possible outcome but evaluating them in terms of maximum risk as well, deciding whether it is worth it or not, whether to stop when risk reaches a certain point, and so on. In one of the very rare articles on medical decision analysis, Jerome Kassirer remarked in 1975 that "good decision-makers should achieve better results on the average than those who have a predetermined pattern of response for each class of clinical problems." But he also says that the decision-making that characterizes most clinical problems is unstructured, mainly because the explicit approach found in decision analysis has not yet gained a foothold in medicine.

To my knowledge, there have been only a very few attempts to apply decision analysis to medical decision-making. All of them appeared in English-language surgical texts and various medical journals. To date there has certainly been no systematic study of the problem, nor is the international medical community even aware that it is a problem. For anyone familiar with decision analysis, it is increasingly evident that doctors should adopt it in everyday practice.

Utilities and Preferences

As a nonmathematician, I am dazzled by the analysis of preferences in uncertain situations Batteau and Marciano set forth. In the framework of utilities or values, which can be described for the "rational" player, the assessment of a given decision-maker's attitude to risk can be very detailed. Risk aversion or a preference for certain kinds of gambles can be analyzed as the player shifts his position according to whether the gamble looks like a "sure thing" (with nothing to lose).

These studies show that what I have outlined about determining and evaluating risks is insufficient. It appears, in fact, that "objective risk" is not what moves the decision-maker. Objective and empirical research, opinion polls, a study of various mathematical operations with known results have allowed decision theorists to classify scales of preference reflecting profound individual differences in dealing with risk. Financial risk for business executives is the usual source of examples. Here we can define a preferred outcome all "players" will agree on, although this does not necessarily mean they will adopt it as an objective. Preferences for gambles with a positive or negative skew (a skew is an uneven distribution of probabilities along the utility continuum) have been charted, as well as complex curves such as the way the attitude to risk varies with the size of the stakes.

In constructing decision trees, each node must be assigned not only a probability—objective or subjective—but also a "preference." A flawless decision analysis under uncertainty can thus lead to quite dissimilar decisions (something we see happening every day).

We should add that for the mathematician the very existence of a structure of preferences under uncertainty presumes that the decider is able to make a complete inventory of possible choices and establish a complete preordering of his preferences. Each of two possible results thus opens onto a possible choice in a stable fashion. This is where the decider's consistency comes into question with regard to preferences. Consistency is an indispensable quality, although it still does not necessarily imply that a decider's evaluation of utilities is rational.

The latter is even more complex than it first seems. Theorists have worked on the existence of multicriteria choices—in other words, cases where utilities vary according to irreducible criteria (politics, economics, ethics). They have devised rules for the composition of individual choices with multiple criteria. We will not go into them, but the fact they exist emphasizes a crucial problem in medicine, bringing us back to the question of finalities. We have seen that even if we assume the decision-maker takes these choices into account (which would be ideal), each physician weighs them differently, without the help of decision theory's guidelines.

The body of work resulting from decision analysis is undoubtedly of great interest to doctors. Physicians are categorized by their preferences, as we have already seen. Yet we can at least expect them to relate their preferences specifically to the idea of maximum service to patients. A gambler risks nothing but his money. A doctor gambles with the health and welfare of others, and there can be no laxity in his preferences. Moreover, mathematics does not allow a preference to be stated until the decision-maker has made a complete inventory of possible choices and established priorities. Otherwise a statement of preference can only be inconsistent. This might be all right in a game of chance, but it is not acceptable when outlining a course of therapy.

There is more to it, as we have seen, since preferences are not synonymous with utilities or values. In the final analysis a physician should assign each node in his decision tree a utility rating and justify it by weighing the multiple criteria involved in the decision. They are all irreducible even though they all center on the patient's best interest: quantity of life, physical quality of life, benefits or physiological consequences, changes in physical appearance and image in the eyes of others.

My reading of decision theory (which I recognize as mine alone, the outgrowth of my personally slanted inquiry and my ignorance of mathematics) leaves me with mixed feelings. On the one hand, I see my overwhelming inadequacy, the way dare I say all doctors are unequal to the task they assume. Even if we put aside the problem of finalities, what do we know about the consistency of probabilistic judgments, making decision trees, structuring preferences logically in the case of a multicriteria choice? What are we to think of scales of individual preferences? Is it acceptable for a patient to be steered toward a therapeutic strategy representing nothing except his physician's preferences? Everything leads us to believe (and I would say I believe) that this scale of preferences is not clear to the doctor instrumenting it. These few questions show that even my brief survey of decision theory provokes some staggering thoughts.

And still medicine goes on, makes progress, has successes. There are doctors whose students and patients acclaim them as masters of the art of healing. What that really means is that their sequence of decisions is the right one: they foresee the course of events with accuracy, correctly determine the preferences and utilities linked with multicriteria choices, make decisions under risk with the fullest awareness of their patients' interest. Teachers of mine who had never been taught how to make decisions were skilled technicians and great strategists nonetheless, consistent, rational, and able to understand and defend the best interests of the very different individuals who placed their trust in them.

We know that men like these, artists like these, do exist, which is reassuring. There have always been great strategists, great deciders, long before Pascal, Montmort, Bernoulli or Borel thought of translating decision-making into mathematical terms.

However, we cannot rely on the chance appearance of exceptionally gifted physicians. There are never more than a handful of them at any one time, while the majority of doctors, as Kassirer points out, respond to a wide variety of situations with predetermined reactions. No one who has been seriously ill or has had a very sick child can see a comparison between decisions about industry and about a human life. There *are* decisions affecting the community as a whole; they can have grave consequences. And nothing would prevent the community as a whole, if it one day becomes rational, from trying to find better ways to recruit and train its decision-makers. Yet nothing seems to equal the intensity of the encounter between a human being in fear of his own or a loved one's life and another human being whose job it is to choose, under uncertainty, the best—or least bad—path through a virtually impenetrable thicket of biological, psychological and material possibilities. On one side is a patient offering what he holds most precious (at times we may value a project or goal more than our lives, but not when we are sick). On the other is a man, nothing more, with the heaviest of responsibilities, the mission of leading his patient through the welter of chance toward the best possible outcome. How can we refrain from using our full potential, considering the tools medicine has at its disposal today?

It is up to the community at large, of course, to decide. It can have a corps of cool technicians with a truly gifted healer appearing once in a great while, or it can have the best doctors possible, providing the best possible care. It can rely on scientific progress in medicine—which will continually be made, slowly reducing uncertainty for future generations of doctors. Or it can demand the utmost of today's physicians, a skillful blend of the art of medicine with available technology.

This book can only make suggestions, not choices, so I will stop here. But a few thorny questions remain to be discussed.

CHAPTER VIII

Finalities in Medicine

IN THE LAST CHAPTER I stressed the difference between finalities, goals and objectives, and how decision-making invariably implies determining an ultimate frame of reference. While medical ethics is not my main subject, it is almost impossible to avoid discussing it. To do so would be absurd, precisely because of the sense of crisis now reigning in medical ethics. The medical profession, and each individual doctor, should have a code to refer to in case of doubt. This is one of the most difficult subjects imaginable, affected by differences in religion, philosophy, desires, neuroses; various conceptions of individual and collective destiny; imperatives, prohibitions, laws, and who knows what else?

Furthermore, the problem of medical ethics cannot be discussed outside its social and cultural context, despite the fact that it has to do with intangible codes of behavior. The marked weakening of certain values and traditions now being seen in Western civilization, as well as the added measure of freedom, mobility and information this civilization affords the individual, are at the root of the crisis. To my mind, the fact that this situation has arisen is to the credit of a civilization that has simultaneously developed science, technology, and humanism. The Judeo-Christian and Greek traditions we inherited have given rise to a parallel growth in technological skill and humanist thinking, resulting in dynamic contradictions. Other cultures, which have fostered neither, are now trying to make us feel guilty about our accomplishments. If we give in, it will be an incontrovertible sign of our loss of self-esteem, confidence and identity. It is up to professionals to meet the challenge, to disseminate, defend and develop the values they embody. Although a "solution" to the modern crisis in medical ethics would not eliminate any of the concrete conflicts I hope to define later, we must begin by discussing this crisis and possible approaches to it.

Ethics in Medicine

Two articles appearing in the same issue of *The New England Journal of Medicine,* one by Carleton Chapman and the other by Thomas Ballantine Jr., very aptly illustrate the problem, showing how far behind physicians are in this area and what the consequences are for the public. They emphasize that even today the major works in English on medical ethics are basically concerned with relationships between doctors, rather than doctor-patient relationships. There are historical reasons for this, having to do with the need to organize the medical profession as it slowly gained recognition for its unique mission of healing. But the lag has now become a serious matter; some people are claiming medicine is a commerce like any other. It is simple enough to demonstrate that this is not at all the case, that most doctors behave according to unwritten rules that define service to others as the finality of their actions. Still, it would be preferable to have it clearly stated, recorded, taught. The Hippocratic oath—in France, the only text in the medical profession exposing students to this vast set of problems—is quite insufficient. The French code of ethics is more explicit, but still inadequate. There have been proposals in the United States to assign medicine the same status as any business, to allow competition and advertising (in hope of lowering health care costs). In France there have been suggestions to abolish the Ordre des Médecins, which would do away with its power to censure practices allowable under the law but ethically questionable. This is another way of saying that the doctor's job is no different from the industrialist's, the merchant's, the veterinarian's, or the railroad man's. They are all respectable callings, but in no way imply a moral duty to serve others, put their interest first and be ready to advise them in the most difficult situations.

Allowing medicine's mission to be degraded in this way would be unforgivable, and those now blinded by partisan and circumstantial considerations would be the first to protest if doctors did not place stricter moral demands on themselves than most people do. Thus, as Chapman suggests, a modern code of medical ethics should be written, no matter how hard it may be to reach a consensus, and it should be taught in medical schools. He stresses that such a code would mean attaining not only a level of competence that fulfills legal expectations but also a level of excellence, guaranteeing that each patient would receive the best possible care.

Ballantine presents the idea a bit differently, showing that medical ethics must be considered as higher than the law, while not above the law. He concludes (and doctors and future patients should thank him for doing so) that physicians should follow an ancient principle: noblesse oblige. He explicates the term as "benevolent and honorable behavior considered to be the responsibility of persons of high birth or rank." He gives the definition of "benevolent" as "kindness, charity and a desire to promote the welfare of others." Doctors are obviously not of high birth, but a high rank is conferred with a medical degree: the right to care for others. Ballantine calls for "moral regeneration," with the principle of noblesse oblige applied to the entire medical profession.

Medical Associations

Theoretically, an ethical code would not include penalties, as the law does, but only rewards in the form of a silent inner pride for those who adhered to it rigorously. However, medical practice shares much common ground with the law, and more important, there are never too many safeguards when the life and welfare of human beings are at stake. For this reason, it is good, wise and reassuring to have a body of doctors elected by their peers to deliberate on rules and regulations as medicine grows more complex, giving doctors a means of regulating their behavior from inside the profession, in the patient's best interest. The law is not enough. All it requires is that minimal rules be observed. What is more, it is fallible. We need a medical association to protest against internment of political prisoners in mental institutions, for example; to defend staunchly the principle of confidentiality against all sorts of encroachments. Having a medical association also protects the principle of the patient's free choice of a doctor, an absolutely minimal requirement in terms of the patient's basic rights, but more crucially in terms of his chance to find the doctor he instinctively realizes he will be able to work with and trust.

Consumer Research

Sociologists and physicians might think that well-conceived and correctly conducted polls could provide us with an indispensable parameter: a knowledge of what the consumers of our services want. And as far as I know, we do not have any information like this. It would be wonderful to have and probably not hard to gather. Yet I cannot help being skeptical about how helpful such research would be, simply because my personal experience has shown me how extraordinarily variable patients' demands are. Whoever had to synthesize the information would have the impossible job of averaging out completely categorical and sometimes contradictory opinions. The researcher would have to interview people according to age, education, religion, income and political opinion, or else end up with what information specialists call "background noise." And they would find that these parameters, not to mention the influence of personal or family experience, have a profound influence on how people see medicine and what they think it should be.

But it would also become clear—and all my observation leads me to insist heavily on this point—that there is no comparison between the way sick people and well people view finalities in medicine. By the sick I mean anyone who has, or believes he has, a serious illness, producing anxiety and fear for one's life or bodily functioning. When my book *Conquering Cancer* came out in the United States, critics unanimously attacked the passage where I questioned whether every patient ought to be told the truth, even when it is devastating ("You have two months to live. Here's what you will probably go through, and we won't be able to do anything about it"). In the United States a great many doctors do have a policy of telling the truth, and all kinds of patients' rights groups demand it. Still, I cannot help noticing that in patients with a very serious illness (the kind whose successive roles in the human mind Susan Sontag illustrates in *Illness as Metaphor*), only a tiny minority demands to know the truth. Then what they want to hear is the general diagnosis, sometimes the overall prognosis, never the prognosis in detail. The more severe the illness becomes, the less curiosity they display. I have finally formed an opinion about this lack of curiosity. It is not that the patients are unaware of the diagnosis—most often they have strong suspicions, at the very least—nor are they unaware of what may happen. They simply do not want to hear the hard words that might destroy whatever slim, perhaps irrational but still invincible hope they have: there has been a mistake; a miracle, science, magic, or chance will save them. Hope helps keep them alive, thinking about the future. Without hope for the future, life is unbearable, except perhaps for saints or heroes.

So I do not think polling the public would be any help. But what if doctors were polled? I am not sure whether it has been done. It would be fascinating to have an intelligent, rigorous, complete questionnaire, with not just a sampling of doctors responding (which would be very hard to select) but the whole country's medical profession. This would give us a mean, and it would be most instructive to compare the answers from each age group, medical specialty, religious affiliation, geographical location, social background. The answers would concern not only euthanasia and its variants, abortion and contraception, but also the lengths to which therapeutic measures should be carried and under what conditions (age, life expectancy, diagnosis; the opinions of the patient, the family and specialists); the medical view of amputation, very disabling illnesses, various sexual dysfunctions; and many other questions.

We could not expect a poll like this to reveal a norm. The diversity of opinions and practices might even be dismaying, since it would emphasize to what extent chance reigns in medicine, insofar as a given patient cannot know his doctor's framework of finalities (unless some kind of nonverbal channel allows doctor and patient to communicate and gain each other's trust). Yet even if we did not expect agreement, or a general rule, to emerge from the poll, what a fascinating picture of today's medical community it would give us! And how vitally interesting it would be to compare our results with those from countries near and far. I see this as a wonderful, if formidable, job for an international organization such as UNESCO.

With the results of this research in hand, two of the most difficult questions would have to be addressed. First, should we work toward establishing a homogeneous ultimate framework of finalities? Should we instate a moral code? Or should we let diversity reign—that is, make no attempt to control the different viewpoints, except with a code of ethics forbidding flagrant abuse and imposing certain imperatives?

Second, should we allow the individual doctor's or the medical profession's finalities or final causes to take precedence over the patient's? This happens when the patient does not know all the factors at work in his case, or when his lack of experience prevents him from accurately evaluating possible "gambles." I will try to address these questions; it is easy to see there are no unequivocal responses.

Individual, Species, Stock

It is nothing new to say that the interests of the individual do not coincide with those of the species. There are several points of conflict. The species is not interested in those of its members no longer able to reproduce or raise young. Humankind alone has tried to forestall this decline and lengthen individual life. If a human decides to procreate after a certain age, there are additional risks for the offspring, since chromosomal abnormalities occur more frequently with age.

In this conflict the doctor naturally sides with the individual. He must be aware of it. Tradition can incite parents to throw defective newborns off cliffs, as the Spartans did, but it has nothing whatever to do with the practice of medicine. It is not the doctor's role to kill or sterilize individuals for eugenic reasons. If doctors were to do so, they would not only be guilty of abominable crimes, but would also immediately and irrevocably lose their standing as physicians. Eugenic murder is absolutely incompatible with medicine. I believe doctors must stifle any inclination to serve the interests of the species if they in any way compromise the interests of the individuals who place their trust in a physician. In the long run, genetic engineering will resolve some aspects of the controversy by ensuring both individual health and the health of the genetic stock. For that reason, I believe it is inevitable. Until then, if any unfortunate society sides with the species (which has happened in recent memory), then let them train killers, but let us make sure no one takes them for doctors.

Individual and Society

Here the conflict is more immediately apparent from a medical point of view, and a doctor is frequently tempted, in all good conscience, to side with society. As we enter hard times, these conflicts will become far more acute than we ever imagined, even allowing for the forms of social assistance that have radically transformed life in our societies. There was once a consensus on the need for social services. They are now held in place by inertia, and the legal system's concern for equality before the law. In the future we may see brutal competition between society's productive members and consumers of social services. I am not talking about the unemployed, who are potentially productive and whose fate depends on economic and political measures outside my sphere. I am talking about the elderly and the chronically ill. I am talking about patients whose lives can be prolonged by a few years—and who want them to be—through costly treatments, with no hope of ever working again. I am talking about old people who once would have died within months of one of the many pathological disorders modern medicine treats as a chronic condition. A patient comes to mind: an eighty-nine-year-old woman who came to us saying she had breast cancer, that she wanted "real" therapy and hoped we would not consider her age a drawback.

Economic responsibilities of this kind will become considerably greater in the coming years. They will weigh more and more heavily on the productive members of society, who will pay higher and higher taxes to support social services. As this happens, we must expect more or less overt, more or less conscious pressure will be put on doctors. Of course we will never be told outright not to fight so hard for patients over seventy. But from my point of view concerning medicine's finalities, two possibilities are to be feared. First, the productive segment of society might reach a sort of tacit consensus that there is nothing wrong with letting the old or chronically ill (one's own relatives excepted, of course) "go peacefully." Second, some physicians might quite innocently be won over to this viewpoint, meaning they would be considering the interests of society (no matter how slightly) when establishing their therapeutic strategy.

I have no idea how the doctors and well people among my readers, or political leaders who define society's overall trends, will take these remarks. As a private citizen, I am aware of the pressing economic issues connected to finite resources. But because of all I have experienced and felt through the years with patients coming to me for help, regardless of their age, condition, life expectancy and finality, I will not budge on this point. Not countering this trend, no matter where it originates, would negate thousands of years of tradition, betray charity and humanity, spiritual and rational values. Apparently contradictory values do exist, and balancing them is the art of governing. As a citizen I use my vote to express my choices, and as a witness to history I deplore human society's orientation toward the welfare state. As a doctor, however, I am lock, stock, and barrel behind those who want a longer life. That cannot be haggled over. In the future some politicians or administrators may have the power to reduce my clinical budget. But they will never get me to do it for them. I hope that all physicians will do the same, to preserve what is essential, their status as a human resource against sickness, the avatar of fate. This is the role they have accepted. They have the honor of defending it against interference, attacks, and ridicule, and forgiving such tactics. I do not believe this is off my subject. What good is a good decision-maker if he has not decided whom he serves?

Individuals and Families

Let us be more specific about whom the physician serves. I do not intend to go into the sometimes sordid family conflict that may flare up when there is an illness in the family. I want only to discuss those cases in which family members claim they understand the patient's best interest better than the patient does. We must often concur, especially when a child is involved (though still reserving judgment, since children are people too and some parents can be abusive, self-centered or irrational). I will leave this very delicate problem to pediatricians. Certain choices should probably also be left up to the family when the patient is senile; if necessary, however, the doctor should still protect the patient's inalienable individual rights.

In some cases, though, a perfectly competent patient is kept in the dark about his health problems and his own future. This is an extremely perplexing situation. It starts with a family member making an appointment, bringing the patient's records and a letter from the original doctor. "You mustn't tell him the truth, he wouldn't be able to take it," the relative says. Or else "Be sure not to prescribe radiation therapy, he might figure out what he has." I have already stated my reservations about telling the truth when an illness is very serious. But that does not mean a doctor and members of the family should be allowed to make a pact to treat an adult as if he were a child or mentally deficient. If radiation therapy could help save the patient's life or promise lasting improvement, would there be any valid reason to withhold it? And what are the real reasons behind the family's request? The request may indeed be legitimate, based on a correct evaluation of the situation. There *are* patients who "couldn't take it" if they learned they were seriously ill. For them the truth is worse than their illness. Their families want to protect them from medical sadism or simple blundering.

If the doctor agrees with the family after examining and talking to the patient, it is not difficult to provide the best of care while concealing the diagnosis. But it is indispensable to examine and talk to the patient first. Sometimes the family unconsciously desires silence because they, not the patient, would find the atmosphere unbearable if the truth were told. Every doctor has seen happily married couples refuse to talk about it when one of them has cancer and they both know it. It is as if the patient would be excluded from the world of the living if they admitted it. This is happening less and less often, fortunately. To avoid a painful situation, the family ask that the truth be covered up. The patient is deprived of his freedom and autonomy, and often some of his tools for fighting his illness. He is more easily upset by unpleasant side effects when he does not know the reason for the treatments, or what they can do for him.

I do not claim to have solved this delicate problem with its infinite nuances. But it may be useful to ask doctors to think about it, as well as all those who accuse doctors of denying them their rightful death, while they themselves deny the illness of their loved ones.

Who Is Sick?

Here the question is not whom we serve but how to serve. Certain decisions on therapeutic strategies must be presented differently to a college professor, a factory worker or a career soldier. They have different perceptions of illness, pain and fate; of what will happen if they have to stop working; and so on. It is also obvious that besides professional differences there are much more profound ones influencing the way a patient will take the news and experience his treatment. Among these are religious faith and its intensity, philosophical opinions, temperamental differences. Some people are weak-willed and others dauntless; apparently spineless souls can turn out to be spirited, brave, helpful to those in need, while domineering types can fall apart. I wish we could get right to the bottom of our patients' psyches, evaluate their real attitude toward death, their anxiety, how they feel about losing part of their body or changes in their physical image. I wish we could know what they have felt when similar things happened to people close to them, as well as how they will "use" their sickness in dealing with themselves and their family.

I would not go so far as to state that crucial therapeutic choices are not and should not be influenced by the patient's personality. Decision-making has certain logical requirements. But medicine does not simply work against nature. It works *with* the patient, or sometimes against him (that is, to counterbalance any irrational tendencies or misinformation getting in his way), and we do not need game theory to see that every strategy is modified by the patient's imposing and inevitable emergence as a partner. If the points I discussed above seemed to suggest that medicine is an abstract game, let us now return to reality. To be effective, the physician's choices must account for uncertainty in nature and the patient's psychology, his resources, what he willfully hides and what he cannot express, his symbolic and semantic systems.

In other words, a doctor must learn to be a keen psychological observer. His work gradually teaches him this; a great deal of the physician's experience, as much or more than the experience of illness itself, is how other people deal with illness. But professional skill is not enough. Reflection, reading, remaining open to other areas of experience and knowledge, the silent observation of true teachers, and probably personal brushes with illness are necessary as well. Then and only then does a physician become a good decision-maker. And whether he is a country doctor or a departmental head at a great medical center, he is a true practitioner of the medical arts.

Medicine and Death

By now it ought to be clear that one of medicine's major finalities is serving individuals, "against" the interests of the species, society, and the family if need be; and that one condition of effectiveness in this area is the doctor's psychological finesse, his ability to recognize, if not "read," the patient's personal characteristics, at least those with some bearing on the triple alliance against the patient.

A point we have not discussed is what kind of care we should offer. The medical community has divergent interpretations of this decisive issue, to say the least.

During their final days Generalissimo Franco and Colonel Boumedienne were subjected to heroic measures for what were obviously not purely medical reasons. The doctors treating them in the terminal stages of their illness had surrendered autonomy and ethical judgment to become no more than technological tools in the hands of the powerful. Giving in to these considerations is always disastrous.

On the other hand, there are doctors who practice euthanasia, not passively but actively. They kill their patients when there is no longer a reasonable hope of saving them, or of keeping them alive in acceptable physiological condition. I can understand why those close to a patient in certain kinds of unbearable situations would ask a doctor to help a patient die, simply to put an end to his suffering. But it appears that there are also patients who are not even in pain and wish to die because they have learned "nothing more can be done." I have never come across one, so I have been spared some unpleasant discussions; I would have turned them down. This is why:

One reason is uncertainty about the facts. Every doctor has seen either unexpected rallying from what was thought to be a terminal situation, or else temporary improvement no one had expected, which gave the patient great relief from physical and/or mental suffering, allowing time for spiritual or material problems to be settled. Preventing this from happening would weigh heavily on a doctor's conscience.

A second reason, perhaps less direct, concerns how much trust patients could have for a doctor who practiced euthanasia. While France's newspapers were full of controversy over proposed legislation that might sanction euthanasia under certain conditions, my hospital admitted a woman who was quite obviously beyond help. She had come a great distance by ambulance. Had we been consulted, we would not have advised her to come. But her first concern was to make sure we did not practice euthanasia (she asked the nurses and ambulance attendants; she was afraid to ask a doctor). The answer is we do not. We gave her what we considered the appropriate treatment. Feeling better, she had a long talk with one of us and then the night nurse, and afterwards went peacefully to sleep. I have seen so many patients fight with tremendous energy, some of them winning, others not. I have seen so much gratitude in their eyes, their gestures, for what they knew was our determination to do everything possible for them, that I can hardly imagine their dismay, their terror if they thought for one moment we might kill them off while they were still fighting, even if it was the final struggle. And I know that many patients who came to us in a critical situation would not have done so if we practiced euthanasia.

A third reason is readily apparent. There might be abuse, meaning mistakes. If active euthanasia were legalized, who could be sure it would never be misused in an ultimately curable case or one that might go into a long remission?

There is a final reason. So far no one has been able to reduce human life to the sum of its chemical components. There is a world of difference between the morphological organization of fossilized protobacteria and the simple coacervates the Soviet biologist Oparine suggests existed in the primitive ocean. There is no proof that the number of "events," in the physicist's sense of the word, the earth has seen since its condensation is equal to the number of mutations required to get from protozoan to human, if these mutations were simply a cumulation of chance occurrences. No one knows when, how or why matter began to undergo the transformations that would endow it with consciousness, in the form of the human brain. Nor when, how or why DNA appeared, to be transmitted in an unbroken chain over billions of years. In his *Princeton Gnosis,* Raymond Ruyer remarks that DNA means what is alive has never died. I, for one, do not feel I have the right to break this chain deliberately. To the dismay of some of my Catholic, Protestant and Jewish friends, I am a convinced agnostic, since as far as I can see the problem of primal causes is insoluble. But this only makes me more disposed to consider any threat to life, including active euthanasia in terminal cases, as a crime against humanity, and I think all doctors ought to agree. Let others do otherwise, if they can. But it ought to be clear that physicians can never under any circumstances kill.

The distinction between active and passive euthanasia should not be thought of as specious. Sometimes life is maintained only by artificial means, as long as a machine pulsates or a transfusion drips. Life would have ended long ago without these support systems, and will stop once they are withdrawn. Then nature has already handed down its verdict, even if an electroencephalogram still shows brain activity. Furthermore, the patient is completely unaware. It is absurd and inexcusable for a situation like this to continue. Once it has been diagnosed, what would otherwise become a parody of medicine must be halted.

Often the necessity to relieve unbearable pain or disastrous physiological situations slowly results in a state where passive euthanasia becomes a possibility. Painkillers bring sleep, but become less effective with time. Muscle tension or moaning show the pain has returned, that the patient is conscious of nothing but pain. So stronger doses are given, and little by little the interplay of illness and drugs brings life to a quiet end. To the very last the physician will have tried to give relief, do all he could for the person sleeping beneath an oxygen mask. Would killing him in cold blood do any good for anyone?

Heroic Measures?

France's Order des Médecins recently proposed making a distinction I find very welcome, one I have tried to use for years in my own practice without stating it as such, and which I believe is at the core of medicine's finalities. Oncologists are easily accused of using heroic measures; they are consulted after the surgeon or radiation therapist, and often too late. Rather curiously, however, the accusation frequently backfires, as we shall see. For instance:

After years of dialysis for kidney failure—triweekly, with the usual complications—a transplant is recommended. There is the wait for a compatible organ, the operation, the body's attempts at rejection, sometimes very serious infections linked to the use of immunosuppressive drugs. Then the final rejection, emergency reimplantation of an organ from another donor, more drugs. The patients who request and undergo this sort of treatment are legion. So are the physicians working with them, applying and perfecting the treatment, facing defeat and beginning again. No one in the medical community calls it heroic measures. The same goes for some seriously disabling diseases of the heart or blood vessels, in which medicine perpetuates a precarious, uncomfortable, even agonizing situation, always at the patient's demand.

Then why is oncology singled out? It may have something to do with the fact that for many people cancer has become the modern equivalent of the devil. They are convinced nothing can be done about it. So they are very hard on anyone who does try, and those who do nothing about cancer can rest easy. Yet by not doing anything they ignore reality (the progress which has been made in the fight against cancer) and their patients suffer for it. These physicians—the most outspoken defenders of "white lies"—create the frightful situation where crucial decisions are made in secret, keeping the patient from choosing to rise to the situation and fight. This is a perversion of medical finalities. In cases where I am personally convinced treatment will be successful, some patients who come to us do not share my confident outlook, since they are still under the sway of the diabolical aura surrounding the word cancer.

Many patients tell me they have deliberately chosen to fight, to undergo any treatment necessary, to stand up for themselves. In the process they reveal unsuspected strengths and meet one of the greatest, most significant challenges of their lives. It is not acceptable to deprive people of this experience, this hope, even a chance of being cured (as increasingly happens). Depriving them of it in all good conscience and crying "heroic measures" when therapy is suggested is not a comfortable intellectual situation.

This is where we should be *persistent,* not heroic. Persistence is perhaps the key word in this book, since it expresses the fact that while there are a few therapeutic strategies guaranteed a 100 percent success rate, in other cases nothing but the physician's persistence can produce a favorable outcome. Here a discouraged doctor (to my mind they are mutually exclusive terms) would not succeed. We owe it to our patients to be persistent. They need to have rock-solid confidence that we will be. How many lives have been saved because a cardiac massage was continued long beyond the suggested time limit? Or because a surgeon undertook a long, systematic dissection of tissue, fraught with difficulty, in a patient many of his colleagues would simply have "sewn up"? How many others have been saved by kidney, heart or cancer specialists who did not admit defeat after the first or second relapse?

It might be argued that the line between persistence and heroic measures is a fine one, even nonexistent. Untrue: heroic measures mean continuing a treatment when it offers no possibility of improvement. This is absurd. A new treatment should immediately be started, or if all the possibilities have been exhausted, treatment should be suspended. This is why heroic measures are very rarely used, in reality. Most often it is simply a case of persistent treatment. The confusion is unfair and deadly. If the choice were left up to patients, they would indubitably choose persistence over stopping treatment. I have never, directly or indirectly, found evidence to the contrary.

Prolonging Life

Even though he was a doctor's son, Aristotle oversimplifies the problem of finality in his *Ethics,* saying a physician is not concerned with ends, but only means, since the goal is always the same: curing the patient. It is true that in most cases when we admit a patient with severe and very widespread lesions we try to come up with a winning strategy, not merely a palliative one. In so doing, we know that certain patients will be saved, others merely given a little longer life. Sometimes, too, only a palliative strategy seems reasonable to us, since the disease has progressed to the point where a cure is beyond our power. Once again, how are we to judge? The ideal thing would be to talk openly with the patient, though what he was told would be purely statistical. It would go something like this: "Without treatment, the disease you have takes its toll in an average of three months, with ten months as the extreme. Treatment would give you an average of nine to twelve months, eighteen at the longest. Which do you choose?"

I realize it is a very difficult choice. Yet only once in my career has a patient (an American who consulted me in the United States) told me: "If you can give me a year, I'll take it. I'm not interested if it's only three months." The patient knows he is in danger, does not ask any questions about the prognosis, yet fights and shows his approval of the treatment by complying with it, no matter what it involves. If the treatment is a success, if the patient is not only alive six to eight months later but in better shape, the family and the original doctor begin to approve of our treatment too. If the results are negative and we lose the patient after three or four months, we run a great risk of being accused of using "heroic measures," if not "experimentation." Not always, for a great many families beg us to try everything, even in the most desperate circumstances. But in any case, what does it matter? Except for terminal situations in which treatment should be aimed at simply giving maximum comfort (anything else would be unreasonable and condemnable) the outcome is undecidable. Only an attempt at treatment can show us whether improvement is possible.

In the case of even partial success, the patient's only alternative is pursuing therapy. Then there is a quantitative question: in incurable cases today, what is the maximum acceptable prolongation? In weighing an answer, the effects of treatment, which vary from case to case, must be taken into account. I will give no answer. I wish only to call attention to the danger that a doctor might decide instinctively, drawing on his image of health, his more or less conscious abhorrence of illness, and so on. The problem deserves to be pondered in the framework of an in-depth study of medicine's finalities and thus of patients' needs and desires. Let me only say that a patient always senses it when treatment is suspended, and is always very upset. Stopping treatment, like cutting down on time spent with a patient in deteriorating condition, is a way physicians unconsciously hurt their patients. Yet in our profession awareness is a minimum requirement if we are to serve effectively and fully.

Taking Risks

There is no effective treatment, especially in the area of medicine dealing with uncertain outcomes, which does not involve the possibility of complications, which can be fatal and are often serious or irreversible in terms of functioning. Immunosuppressive drugs mean that transplant patients are permanently prey to potentially serious or fatal infections. Anti-cancer drugs can damage the bone marrow, sometimes the kidneys or lungs. Sometimes surgery removes a deadly tumor only at the price of postoperative shock so serious the patient hovers between life and death for days. Delegating the choice to the patient, as often happens in the United States, where an "enlightened consent" form must be signed or rejected, is only a partial solution; a patient can never fully grasp all the elements at work in a case. Furthermore, he often turns to the doctor for help and asks him to make the decision. The doctor must therefore be ready and willing to evaluate this delicate situation. As we have seen, decision-making under risk is no easy thing in absolute terms. In medical terms it is even more delicate, and the decider's disposition must not affect it. The "daredevil" physician is a public menace. So is the overcautious doctor, giving his personal peace of mind priority over the patient's chances of survival.

There are cases in which great risks must be taken, or else failure is certain. In others even a slight risk is inadmissible, if, for instance, there is a good chance of a cure without additional treatment. The only parameter guiding this kind of decision is the patient's best interest, his life, his functional wholeness. These must be evaluated with consistency, and a doctor must be wary of his own motives. Several years ago when I suggested to an American thoracic surgeon that we try intradermal injections of BCG on lung-cancer patients in order to see how much time could be gained, he answered, "I wouldn't be able to put my patients through skin ulcers that could take several days to heal."

One day a surgeon sees a young man in urgent need of a kidney transplant. The man's sister has agreed to be a donor and tests show she is very compatible. This is an ordinary enough situation. After all the tests have been done, the surgeon has second thoughts and refuses to perform the operation. What if the sister's remaining kidney were endangered later in life? The surgeon feels noble, going against established and effective practice and causing the brother and sister the greatest distress in the process. Serving others really is not so simple.

The Irrational Patient

However, going along with the patient's wishes does not always mean serving his best interests. Some patients will not consent to an operation that represents their only chance of survival, or refuse a therapy with unpleasant side effects. They will go from doctor to doctor, multiplying their chances of finding one who "understands" them and through an error of judgment, or out of weakness, offers them exactly what they are looking for. This is obviously no way to serve patients. But convincing them is difficult, and I do mean convincing, not merely contradicting them. Some will complain about authority figures, claim they are not being listened to, and that will be the end of the conversation. The doctor's duty then is to do everything possible to allow the patient to overcome his aversion or his fear, to give him examples, time to think things over, if need be to have him meet other patients with the same disease who would be willing to share their experiences. Even so, there is no guarantee of success.

Who Is Providing Care?

Being a good doctor is easier said than done, and it would be very wrong to infer from this book that I believe I am always equal to the situation. Every doctor has his own personal makeup, his moods, beliefs, prejudices and neuroses. When he has not neglected thinking about the profession's finalities, he also has his own opinion of them. Further, he has what I might call his whims. Right away he finds some patients less likeable than others because they are too talkative or quiet or spineless or sure of themselves, because they are too resigned or too inquisitive, because they brought four vocal people along to their appointment.

A good doctor must know how to deal with all this, reconnoiter the situation, make the right choices, find a way to help the patient accept them, minimize the trauma of seeing a doctor, of what the doctor has to say. A doctor must keep himself from seeking any psychological gratification, or rather find gratification only in the feeling of having reached the best possible decision, through the best interpretation of possible outcomes and finalities. A difficult exercise; it keeps one humble, watchful, and thinking critically, rather than overconfident and self-satisfied. It demands a slow reworking of one's character, so that unproductive feelings or judgments will not interfere with professional behavior, make it less up to standard or less effective. This effort at self-improvement has to do not with an individual physician's worth, but with the greatness of the profession.

One or Several Finalities?

It might be presumed, as I have already said, that the finalities of medicine vary greatly from one doctor to the next, resulting in different courses of action, different goals in similar situations, thus different choices. Even if we were able to minimize these differences, other divergences would remain. They stem from the wide variety of beliefs and experiences doctors have in many areas. The public must simply put up with this state of affairs. The fact is that in a given situation three different doctors will give three different opinions.

If there were a group of researchers insane enough to attempt a detailed codification of medical behavior, in hope of protecting us from the results of this diversity, they would subsequently have to find either a totalitarian regime able to enforce the code or else obedient physicians. In either case there would be an enormous risk of having medicine become dry, inhuman, depersonalized. Only as a free individual can a doctor serve effectively. We must accept the drawbacks this involves and staunchly defend our freedom. The patient must also be free to consult several physicians if he feels a need to do so, and form his own opinion. In some countries a patient can consult only the specialist assigned to his case. A travesty of medicine is the inevitable result.

The finalities of medicine have not been precisely formulated. Of course it would be good to have physicians' thoughts on the subject, but all sorts of other governmental and professional organizations should speak out as well. After all, medicine serves everyone. It is sometimes criticized, justly or unjustly; past and future consumers of health care should also view medicine as food for deep and dispassionate thought.

But perhaps a few points can help us gauge how crucial and complex the problem is. And how the prodigious growth of technology may keep the public, as well as doctors, from seeing that all medical practice has to rest on a foundation of fellowship. To achieve this kind of relationship with others, doctors must grow throughout their lifetimes to attain a vision of society and humanity that would make this fellowship natural, make sure doctors automatically and permanently follow the principle of noblesse oblige.

This crisis will not be resolved by the proliferation of lawsuits, by checks on medicine's technical activity, or especially by diminishing doctors' liberty. We must forge for our societies the most responsible and devoted medical corps possible and focus our attention on the quality of the men and women who will be invested with the mission of caring for and curing others. This effort is indispensable if we want decisions made on the technical level to be the best decisions in terms of service to human beings.

CHAPTER IX

Improving Decisions, Improving Decision-Makers

At this point it ought to be clear that in every country where individualized medicine thrives, the quality of medical care could be markedly improved without any change in the health-care system or any additional scientific progress. It would simply be a matter of eliminating faulty decision-making, losing therapeutic strategies, inconsistent choices. I would not venture to say exactly how much of an improvement we could count on, but from a certain point of view that is not very important.

Medicine has no room for anything but excellence. A two-pronged effort would give rapid results. First, medicine should make use of what decision analysis has to teach. Medical students should become acquainted with the set of problems and solutions it proposes. Second, each doctor should have the principles of medical ethics at the center of his thinking, his inner life. He should be constantly aware of the great questions and challenges put to medical ethics every day in our changing times.

Is it worth a try? An important question, which potential patients as well as doctors, academic institutions and government agencies will have to answer. For my part, I have come to believe that it is an urgent task, and an impelling one. We must see if our societies are able to identify a major problem of concern to everyone and propose remedies to it.

I have said that medicine is the science of troubleshooting; the same holds true for politics. It is a less exact science, if anything, since the social body is even more complex and less understood than the biological body. And it cannot rely on experimentation. There is one advantage, however: the social body seems less fragile. It tolerates more serious therapeutic errors and compensates for them in some way. But just as in medicine, politics should not be in the hands of the doctrinaire. Politicians should be willing to monitor their mistakes and change course accordingly, accept the idea that they are fallible and that it is nothing to be ashamed of. If all this is true, and since here in France it could hardly hurt for the medical-school curriculum to be revised (the last reform of the curriculum was a disaster), why couldn't we have a reform based on logic instead of demagogy this time around? All we would need is accurate markers allowing us to measure positive or negative results and political measures allowing us to backtrack if necessary. With these idealistic notions in mind, I offer the following suggestions.

Teaching Finalities

Experience has made me see that having a solid ethical frame of reference is a prerequisite for any thinking about the quality of decisions. And I have learned that not only is the medical code of ethics unwritten—with the exception, in France, of the code of deontology—but also that the French medical curriculum contains only one lecture on the subject in a six- or seven-year program. For all sorts of reasons, it is time to change things and familiarize students with the very essence of their future profession. Otherwise the current situation, unsatisfactory in more ways than one, will simply perpetuate itself. The exposure each doctor has to the problem of his profession's finalities is extremely variable, and at least partly left up to chance.

Some doctors have a natural inclination or the philosophical background to cope with finalities. Others, not necessarily worse doctors for it, are more inclined to action than speculation. They evolve reflex behaviors and rarely stop to explore the whys and wherefores. A small minority of doctors are in the wrong line of work, and only intra-professional censure forces them to observe minimum ethical standards. How much more satisfying it would be if each of our future doctors had had to think about the nature of the profession all during his medical studies, with the help of carefully chosen texts: about the nature of his relationship to others, the standards of excellence in the profession, the care he will have to provide all his life for his fellow humans; about ethics and moral considerations in general, their comparative status in various cultures, their place in our own, the controversies they give rise to, and so on.

I was never told as a student that noblesse oblige should be the guiding principle of my behavior, and I am very sorry I was not. It might have changed my life. I found it out only after long years of rough guesses, indifference, learning bit by bit. A doctor must be a person like any other, seeking and finding fulfillment in private life. But in his professional life there can be nothing frivolous. Medicine means serving others.

It took me many years to understand why Alexis Carrel thought doctors should lead a monklike existence, sheltered from worldly cares. I think this was an inappropriate, awkward way of expressing a completely legitimate standard. Doctors who were taught to thoroughly analyze and discuss the ethical implications of their attitudes would set the highest standards for themselves. They would know for certain, and with pride, that they are the helping hand every human being hopes to find when illness strikes.

It remains to be determined who should be in charge of teaching ethics and how it should be done. Since we have no experience in this area, it is difficult to say. It seems to me that students should have the chance to meet representatives of all religious and philosophical movements, and discuss mutual problems with them. But I believe an essential part of the curriculum should be devoted to courses taught by doctors, and the detailed examination of specific cases, with the patients or their families present, if need be. Each speciality would have a special course tailored to its own demands. The atmosphere in which medical decisions are made would be completely transformed. Every technical discussion would be patient-centered; the patient is both subject and object of the discussion. The point would be identifying his best interest, determining how it can best be served and defended.

It follows, then, that medical psychology must also be reworked and rethought. Future doctors need more than a summary of what the various branches of psychology have to teach. They must learn how illness changes or heightens human psychology and what it does to communication. We still have a great deal to learn in this area. Yet as far as I know what has been discovered to date has not been put in any form medical students can use, which is really too bad. This knowledge may not be indispensable to the elaboration of finalities, but it is needed each time these finalities are applied to a specific case.

A possible, if not serious, objection to my proposal is the already crowded curriculum in medical schools. It would be better to keep future doctors in school for an extra year than to settle for the vague understanding of these subjects they are now given.

Aptitude Testing as a Means of Selection

Today competitive tests in math or physics are the primary means used to select future doctors, on the pretext that an understanding of math is essential for the study and practice of medicine (which is patently false) and that it is as good a measurement of intelligence as any other (which is beside the point).

For twenty years now I have been working on a daily basis with small groups of students (assigned to the hospital department I head), carefully observing their reactions. I have often asked myself if all psychological profiles are suited to the practice of medicine, and have concluded they are not, as common sense would also dictate.

I do not intend to compare, let alone influence, the spiritual and philosophical choices of future doctors, useful as it might be to show them how these choices determine their concrete positions, sometimes unconsciously. But we must do away with the myth of the average doctor, abstract, "normal" and neutral, always even-tempered, experiencing only positive emotions as he exercises his profession, and then only to the proper degree. Even if this were considered ideal, a young doctor could never attain it, or even hope to, without being aware of the gap between his own personality traits, psychological profile, disposition and past experience, and the image he has of the profession.

By paying careful attention to students, however, it is easy to see which ones will and which ones will not eventually behave according to the noblesse oblige principle. I am not sure specialists won't think it outrageous of me to assert that the ability to grasp moral problems partly depends on the psychological profile and on behavior. But I am ready to defend my statement.

Young people who appear outlandishly dressed at the bedside of a tired and overwrought patient are not cut out to be doctors. The same is true if they are less than immaculately clean when they have to touch a patient, or if they are short-tempered when their questions are not understood. I would not tend to encourage students to practice medicine if they had poor attendance records and took ten extra days of vacation, or slipped away from work when their supervisor's back was turned. Nor would I want slapdash students who would not care how far off their observations were as long as no one noticed. Nor indifferent ones who would not lose sleep over a patient's distress, or those who answer if you ask them a question, but never ask any themselves and seem totally uninterested. It is often painfully obvious that they have no inkling of the greatness of their potential task, or the existence of finalities beyond their immediate objectives.

Nurses are often the first to register shock at students' behavior, and nurses ought to know. They struggle and work under difficult conditions, are on the floor two hours before doctors get there. Some nurses suppressed the desire to become doctors when they had to go to work at an early age. When they think that in three years a certain student will have a medical degree, will give orders, be taken seriously, they know they would never want to be under his care.

This does not support the idea of selecting students through mathematical aptitude. There is no perceptible correlation between students' ranking in math tests and their behavior. Nor is there any correlation later on between mathematical ability and professional success, effectiveness, or recognition of the noblesse oblige principle.

I do not think it is possible to tell whether an eighteen- or twenty-year-old will be endowed with the moral sense it takes to make a doctor. But after a year or two we should be able to tell if he is never going to have it. Observation, interviews, tests, the opinion of specialists, and patients' evaluations could tell us. When I began my medical studies, first-year students went to a hospital ward every day and examined patients. Later some technocrat decided it was absurd, and now at least two years go by before a future doctor gets anywhere near a patient. But what does it matter, since tests have proved he is a good scientist . . . ?

We could easily demonstrate that all the math needed to practice medicine, even to teach it or contribute to advances in medicine, can always be learned when circumstances require it. The exception is certain laboratory or research careers that do not involve caring for patients. But I know it would not be easy to give up the current methods of admitting medical students, given the force of inertia. The United States may be the only place where there is enough freedom and autonomy, spirit of research and sense of responsibility toward society, for an experiment of this kind to work out or even be tried at all.

Until then, we must settle for knowing that the current selection procedures do not weed out those unfit to be doctors. I am not questioning the level of intelligence of current or future doctors. I am only saying that if they have the right kind of character for their profession—in the fullest sense of the term—and if they also have the necessary breadth of vision and inner richness, it is purely by accident.

Choosing Decision-Makers

Good intentions are obviously not enough. The list of sometimes serious errors committed by physicians full of love for their fellowmen is almost endless. We have seen what an important part correct and safe decision-making plays in a huge area of therapeutics (no matter how new the idea of formalizing it is). Yet we have not even touched the tip of the iceberg. Doctors and medical students are not told that they are decision-makers, often working under uncertainty, or taught that there are techniques available to help them analyze and perhaps improve their decision-making.

Strangely enough, medicine is not the only profession to lag behind in this respect. I know that decision analysis is taught in military academies, but I am not sure that it is a key subject, that mediocre grades in it purely and simply mean an officer will never hold a high command. And what about men and women in government service, or those who court political power?

Everyone acts as if a certificate of good decision-making were handed out as a bonus with a commission or a promotion, as a matter of course. There *are* experts in decision theory, but they are hardly in command positions. In the best and rarest of cases, their advice is solicited, but seldom followed. Most often decisions are based on self-interest or preconceived ideas, or are taken extremely lightly and imposed on those they concern without their consent. Decisions are likewise opposed without the slightest reference to true analysis, especially a simulation of possible outcomes. Instead, ideological arguments are put forward (and in ideologies there is no room for uncertainty).

I do not propose to improve the way human societies are run, but only to draw attention to the problems in decision-making specific to the medical profession. They differ from the needs of military men, economists or politicians, in one important respect: doctors cannot usually meet at length with experts to analyze a problem exhaustively.

Doctors are at once the outside expert and the decision-maker, the analyst and the person in power. They must act quickly, either immediately or after gathering some additional data. Another difference is that they do not give orders, but make suggestions. Some patients quite rightly request a second or third opinion, although I am not at all sure how they eventually make up their minds.

Some doctors even organize teams of specialists working jointly on cases; this is what happens in cancer centers. But it is the doctor who has the administrative power over the team who has the final say. It is high time we focused our attention on the quality of medical decision-making, if we are to keep up with changes in medicine, keep our practice up to the level of therapy now available, and make the most of situations where "scientific" medicine still leaves room for inspiration, or even opens an area heretofore closed off to imaginative inquiry.

I will begin by examining the maximal solution for selecting doctors. I harbor no illusions that it will be adopted in the near future, given the force of inertia, any more than I imagine my remarks on a medical vocation will influence aptitude testing. But I am glad for the opportunity to discuss them here.

There are born decision-makers, as we know from military history, not to mention the achievements of doctors and businessmen. I am talking about instinctive deciders, uninfluenced by the recent developments in decision analysis. It should not be impossible to isolate the traits that make a good decider, even before the fact: the ability to see all the possible outcomes of a course of action (which is far from obvious), logical rigor, consistency in assigning probabilities and assessing risk and acceptable risk, consistency in preferences, and so on. It should not be impossible to test for these traits, although it would not be an absolute criterion for choosing future doctors. Basically it would allow us to identify poor decision-makers, unpredictable or inconsistent ones, the kind that make you wonder what on earth was behind their decisions.

Some people are simply like that. Their gifts may take them far in the arts, mathematics, or any science pursuing certainty.

At all costs they should be steered away from medicine, for all the reasons I have already stated.

As I see it, we ought to be looking for a combination of specific qualities in future doctors: the ability to understand, organize and retain a certain amount of knowledge, keeping in mind that retention is the least important of these, since information can be stored in books or computers or on tape; a medical vocation, by which I mean motivation, the desire to serve and care for patients; emotional stability; the ability to make the best choices under uncertainty. It is too bad that France's universities are not autonomous enough so that here again a single criterion for admission could be changed in a few medical schools. It would take at least ten years to tell if the change was a valid one, but for several decades now the teaching of medicine has been the subject of heated international debate and much experimentation, with no consensus in sight. This comes as no surprise. Over the last thirty years medical knowledge has been replacing itself at an ever-quickening pace. This turnover raises almost insoluble problems for teachers of medicine. Yet once again, while we cannot store the sum of this knowledge at any given moment, we should at least make sure that practicing physicians are not constitutionally indecisive or irrational or both. I do not know if there are already tests that could single out poor decision-makers, but I would venture a guess that the recruitment of airline pilots is more rigorous than medical training in this respect. If I am right, a fairly wide-ranging debate on the subject will be hard to avoid.

Training Decision-Makers

Whether or not admission to medical school is ever based on decision-making ability, it is now possible for doctors to be trained in the techniques of decision analysis so indispensable to today's medicine. It should be a two-part course. The first section would be a survey of decision theory, a required course for all medical students, which would acquaint them with the role this mental process plays in every level of medical practice. Techniques for decision analysis would be explained, as well as the rules governing decision-making under uncertainty.

The course would be aimed at analyzing conventional therapeutic behaviors and the unapparent decisions underlying them; identifying reflex behaviors (in order to curb them), noting how an often totally implicit system of finalities affects decision-making; and showing how decision-making depends both on previous experience and how rigorously data gathering is done in each case. If we could ensure that the general practitioner would think of himself partly as a decision-maker, it would be an important step forward. He would then have a different image of the nature of his responsibilities.

However, specialists and doctors associated with hospitals have the most to do with therapeutic decision-making, as we have already seen. They are the doctors consulted in difficult cases, the ones who have to choose between several strategies every day. Experience has shown that their choices vary from one patient to the next.

At this level, when a physician is trained as a specialist or chief resident, an advanced course in decision-making should be required. It would be part theory and part practice, and passing the final exam would be mandatory. The theoretical part would be taught by specialists in decision theory—mathematicians, perhaps logicians—rather than doctors; their job would be to familiarize the future therapist with the techniques, reasoning, and theories that already constitute a considerable body of organized knowledge. This could be combined with a required course in statistics, sometimes a weak point for doctors who have to evaluate the results of clinical research.

As I see it, the effort involved in working out the problems and exercises a course such as this would entail, the grounding it would offer in the basic principles governing decision-making under uncertainty, would represent an indispensable step toward better-quality medical treatment in that it is no longer admissible to rely on a given doctor's intuition or guesswork when the process can at least partially be formalized and optimized.

My proposal may surprise many people, but it will inevitably become reality. This is obvious to everyone who comes in contact with this field of human endeavor. Decision analysis has repercussions on the technical, scientific and economic functioning of contemporary society.

But along with this theoretical training, where does practical teaching come into the picture? This will involve long hours, over long years, of case-method studies. Each somewhat difficult, somewhat uncertain case should be the subject of group discussion and decision analysis. I imagine that each unit chief would draw up a separate chart of objectives, a decision tree, assigning a probability to each possible outcome (and justifying the way it was calculated), assessing preferences and risks. All this would be done several "moves" in advance so that each senior doctor could write his own strategy. Afterwards they would be compared, a choice reached, and the treatment applied. The results would later be gone over step by step, with reference to the records of the initial decision.

My staff and I hold weekly meetings to review all cases requiring the formulation of a treatment or a change in treatment. Yet, I am sorry to say, we have not gone so far as to formalize the decision-making process. One reason for writing this book is the desire to progress in this area.

A further step would be to have teaching physicians keep a log of decision trees and strategic discussions. This would give us a kind of thesaurus to use in training our students in simulated decision-making, just as airline pilots are taught with flight simulators. Comparing the logs of different medical teams would also be extremely instructive; each decision would refer to a true case history. This would allow us to build data banks and eventually substitute objective probabilities for subjective ones, and penetrate the thought processes of top practitioners, who do not always elucidate the reasons for their success in certain cases.

Even if the decision analyses or algorithms* obtained in this way rapidly became obsolescent, some would remain useful to think about because they contain something inspired, just as I still think about certain winning "gambles" teachers of mine made when I was an intern thirty years ago.

Have there already been attempts to implement this kind of log-keeping? Very few, to my knowledge. Dr. Lagarde of Bordeaux recently organized a conference on decision-making in medicine (which has not yet been held as of this writing). My friend Philip Rubin at the University of Rochester has applied Boolean algebra to the analysis not of concrete cases, but of research strategies used in oncology. Jerome Kassirer of Boston has published an article entitled "The Principles of Clinical Decision-Making: An Introduction to Decision Analysis," coming out of a Clinical Decision-Making Group at Tufts University in 1975.

The author shows how a few examples of applied decision analysis have filtered into the medical literature, without lasting effect. Kassirer's sixteen-page article devotes two and a half pages to a study of football strategy. He then examines the decision tree for a difficult clinical case. The choice was whether or not to operate on a young woman in serious

*An algorithm is a sequence of instructions for solving a problem it is sometimes possible to formulate when decision analysis has been done for a number of similar cases [*Medical Choices, Medical Chances,* pp. 140–41].

condition from a probable abdominal infection. The decision was made not to operate. But two weeks later, as the illness progressed, the results of medical treatments were evaluated, and more testing was done, the situation was reevaluated and the operation was finally performed. Meanwhile, the risks involved in surgery had increased, but the risk of not operating was greater. Kassirer points out that many of the probabilities used in the analysis were arbitrary, or linked to the physicians' "experience," since an exhaustive review of the medical literature did not reveal anything about the risk of various complications or the chances of a nonsurgical cure in patients with a similar complaint.

This remarkable study—which provides an interesting scale of "units" of evaluation of utilities or values, among other things—shows how much the entire medical community, and thus the community of potential patients would stand to gain if case studies like this were published and examined. It implies the creation of a new type of medical literature, reporting not only on clinical research and reducing uncertainty to certainty but also on optimizing strategies under uncertainty. It would be a kind of dictionary of the state of the art. In the very near future it could have a considerable influence on certain kinds of medical endeavor. An intellectual challenge of this magnitude is difficult to resist, and crucial to meet.

Dr. Kassirer mentions some unsolved problems: establishing large bodies of clinical data that could be referred to when assigning probabilities; developing methods for utility assessment compatible with the practice of medicine (doctors and patients alike initially feel uncomfortable with "the arbitrary assignment of numerical values to outcomes such as pain, disability, and death," he says); and also a problem I have not discussed here—estimating a priori probabilities of medical diagnoses. He makes no mention of the art of medicine, except for a brief reference to "good" decision-makers, and he seems to presume that all American medical students are logical, rational beings, all equally attuned to a mathematical or scientific argument and all with the same reasonable attitude toward risk.

If that were true, we would already have noticed it here in France, and in fields other than medicine as well. We would all live in a world governed by logic, goodwill, respect for communal interests . . .

But while Kassirer neglects this aspect of medicine (which fascinates me), he pleads for a rationalization of therapeutic choices. He is far from wrong when he predicts in his conclusion that the widespread application of decision analysis to the everyday practice and the teaching of medicine is forthcoming. How long will it take once the problem has been raised? The question is of interest to sociologists, educators, and future patients.

In this chapter I have tried to give free rein to my imagination, proposing all the measures I see resulting from my earlier analysis and arguments. While I cannot ignore the magnitude of the tasks at hand, I do not think it impossible to transform the practice of medicine. One more way would be selecting doctors according to the new requirements arising from within the profession: defining the service we will give, choosing strategies to that end. This is no way excludes study and work in clinical research, a separate but essential activity, carried on in part by the same people. But that is not my subject here.

My original ambition was to formalize rules for medical practice in order to help raise standards. I was gradually led to consider the problem of the art of medicine as well and amend my working title. It is a difficult problem; I would welcome outside opinions. I will conclude with a discussion of it, aware as I am of my inability to present more than a fragmentary view.

CHAPTER X

The Art of Medicine

THROUGHOUT THIS BOOK I have been trying to give my answer to the old question "Is medicine an art or a science?" Having lived through the rise in therapeutic capabilities, the explanation of an impressive number of physiopathological mechanisms, the discovery of the minute inner working of widely but blindly prescribed drugs such as aspirin or theophylline, I was led to believe that medicine—in everyday practice—would one day become a science. I feel a little ridiculous for having thought so.

The first reason is that I have seen medical artists at work. Some of my teachers gave me unforgettable lessons during my student and intern days. Let me mention only Paul Chevalier among those who are no longer with us, and Robert Worms, Jacques Decourt and Etienne Bernard, who have since retired.

Then too, as I have already said, medicine is best described as the science of troubleshooting, closely related to what engineers do, or mechanics with a flair for tinkering and invention. The only difference is that nature has its own solutions, reworked and refined over millions of centuries of evolution, to the problems of individual survival versus entropy. But we do not know what they are. So medicine must grope its way along, try to get things working again, use its results to reconstruct nature's blueprints with hindsight, and conceive of increasingly operational models. As medicine's ambitions and scope of inquiry have grown, the various biological disciplines have branched off from it. Today they are independent sciences, beginning in turn to contribute to medicine.

The single word "medicine" really denotes a group of radically different activities:

- *Experimental medicine,* the very concept of which gives an idea of Claude Bernard's pioneering spirit, constantly draws on discoveries in biology and also fosters them. It explores the inner workings of a variety of pathological disorders in test tubes and laboratory animals, elaborating therapies to be progressively refined. Experimental medicine sometimes lags behind clinical practice. Research is done to show why or how a specific drug works after it has already been in use for decades. I have no idea how many researchers are working in the experimental field right now. Clearly, however, their work is indispensable and should be encouraged and developed. Experimental medicine has already achieved great things; more advances can be expected in coming years.
- *Clinical research* is another form of medicine I have already discussed. It is not as close to being a "pure" science as experimental medicine is. As evidence one need only cite the low rate of reproducible results from one research team to the next in various clinical trials. The reason for this is that instead of studying standardized populations of genetically similar animals, inoculated at the same age with the same dose of the same therapeutic agent, clinical research works with human beings with spontaneously developed diseases. They are extremely dissimilar, and the same disease will evolve differently from one case to the next. Yet clinical research aims for scientific status. In the process it has learned, for instance, to identify

many sometimes inconspicuous characteristics in patients and divide them into subgroups that are probably more homogeneous.

It has developed a strict methodology for data gathering, administering medication and measuring results. It divides problems up so that each study deals with a single situation, a single question. Finally, it takes care to evaluate its own effectiveness, with rigorous statistical methods intended to eliminate the researchers' subjectivity. Like experimental medicine, clinical research is an irreplaceable tool and an autonomous activity. There is obviously a need for close communication between the two, but it would be wrong to think that clinical medicine merely applies what experimental medicine discovers. In many cases the most useful questions are formulated through clinical observation. In any case, studies are designed in such a way as to exclude any intrusion of the medical art (which would make it impossible to compare the case studies of various researchers). As we have seen, however, this constitutes a separate problem.

• Another step removed from "pure" science is individualized medicine dealing with certainty: spontaneously curable diseases, or illnesses that are always curable with appropriate treatment. I will not say anything further about this except to mention that here skill—the art of medicine—plays an important role. It is at work in the unconscious programming of decisions, since even a certain outcome can be reached by many different routes, varying in length, cost, side effects and discomfort. In short, each decision has a degree of elegance.

Every medical act and every illness leaves its mark. There is an art to minimizing the trauma of a pathological episode, offering comfort and reassurance, a brotherly or (only when absolutely necessary) fatherly presence.

I think I should state once again that far from precluding the art of medicine, family practice requires it. Many of the men and women in family practice are in great demand and are greatly trusted by their patients, and thoroughly deserve to be.

• Finally, there is the branch of medicine that deals with uncertainty, treating serious, chronic, disabling, sometimes (though not always) fatal illnesses. This branch of medicine has grown over the past thirty years and is extending into situations that once always followed a stereotyped course. This kind of medicine—and I include surgery in the definition—ultimately tries to optimize the outcome of each individual case. It is therefore crucial to have rigorous strategic thinking, backed up by best possible assessment of finalities, respecting intangible principles in relation to the individual and his or her life and liberty. While scientific knowledge is indispensable, the sine qua non of success in this area, it takes a back seat to what we justly call the art of medicine, the need for which will always be felt.

Portrait of the Artist

During my residency in Paris, one of my teachers identified an ultra-rare case, the first in France, of sporadic typhus. It was a spontaneous recrudescence, after twenty years, of epidemic typhus the patient had contracted in his youth. Outside the context of an epidemic, the diagnosis was extremely difficult. It was an exciting case because it offered the opportunity to study the relationship between recrudescent and epidemic typhus, to learn whether and how lice might pick up the infection from a sporadic case and spread it to epidemic proportions. The motive was scientific curiosity, but it was not entirely selfless. World War II had just ended, and there was still a chance of typhus outbreaks in Central Europe.

The patient was a Pole who did not understand French very well. He was prostrate after several days of a 104-degree fever.

Everyone was very worked up. Once the diagnosis was certain, a famous bacteriologist from the typhus department brought in a little cage full of laboratory lice and affixed it to the patient's forearm. It was supposed to be left in place for ten days, so the insects' excreta could then be studied to see what was causing the disease, how long it lasted, what it looked like, and if the pathogenic agents were the same as for epidemic typhoid. It was something like a European premiere, promising important and useful knowledge. It was the talk of the staff room. The patient was not in any danger, but was certainly not very chipper. I was doing everything I could for him so that the incubation period would go as smoothly as possible. His wife was upset and depressed; she didn't speak French either.

One morning, two or three days before the advance of science allowed for the removal of the cage, our chief, Dr. Robert Worms, came onto the floor in a mood we had never seen him in. He had slept badly, he was brusque. He said something like "I'm taking that box off of him. I don't care about the experiment. This just isn't right. The man is running a temperature of 104 when Aureomycin would make him better. He doesn't know what's going on. Maybe he fears for his life. And besides, there is just no way to justify prolonging a patient's discomfort." The next day the patient's temperature was back to normal. He was refreshed, aware of what was happening around him. His wife was all smiles, and Dr. Worms was somber. We never talked about the case again.

Doctors have every chance of losing sight of higher finalities, doing a good job when it could have been better, finding unpleasantness more acceptable for others than they would for themselves, or considering a patient's demand exorbitant. Some demands, of course, cannot be met, for several hundred patients at any one time could lay claim to our attention and concern. But it would be more dangerous the other way around, if we were to depersonalize and restrict the relationship with patients. My head nurse sometimes asks me to see a patient one of my coworkers is following. When I tell her just to have the patient make an appointment with my secretary, she invariably tells me he was afraid to ask for himself. If some people find me that hard to approach, I still have a long way to go. The medical artist, as I see him, has achieved utter simplicity, accessibility, transparency. One day I heard Fred Siguier, a great teacher, though not one of mine, say "I don't believe in virtue, but I practice it." And I know that in saying so he was not boasting or exaggerating. The remark came out of years of thinking.

Sometimes it seems to me a patient should be able to go to his doctor the way a child goes to his grandfather, certain that he will be cared for completely, find acceptance, security, in short selfless love, cleansed of any intention to chastise. Just as often I think that would mean treating patients like children, and it would be better for a doctor to show a firm resolve to put his technical know-how, his powers of reasoning at the service of an objective jointly determined by doctor and patient.

No doubt the true medical artist has stopped worrying about it, and instinctively takes the right position. Arriving at the correct solution no longer costs him any effort. I think it was Leon Bloy who wrote that the only real trouble is that we are not saints. We never will be, for good reason. But I have known doctors who may not have been far from sainthood, despite their rough edges. I wonder what this may have to do with disposition and experience. I don't recall having seen it in doctors under fifty, and even after that it is certainly very rare.

Charity is not everything, however. My portrait of the ideal doctor does not stop there. He must also be a talented gamesman. It is admirable how some chess players can calculate several moves in advance and formulate a winning strategy against any defense. Chess masters beat computers. I do not know whether their game is instinctive or discursive, but it really doesn't matter very much. For it means we know there *are* people who, in a one-on-one situation, under uncertainty, know how to play the odds. They are not great mathematicians or scientists. They are basically inspired decision-makers, and sometimes very young. The same is true of top-ranked bridge players. Some situations in bridge have analogies in medicine. There are several possible courses of action. All but one will result in a losing game. The idea is to play a winner's game, not taking useless precautions or wasting precious time in purely academic computations.

Napoleon said that the art of war was simple: it was all in the execution. Only an inspired strategist would say something like that, after a great deal of observation, thought and calculation, imagining drawbacks and possible countermoves. What is more, the strategist must stay on the scene, have a ready supply of replacements, not stick with a losing strategy out of vanity or even adhere to rigid tactics. He must also know how to change objectives, if necessary, rather than give up.

He must be personally responsible, willing to put himself on the line, do the dirty work. If a doctor walks out of a patient's room where the smell is unbearable, leaving his staff or his nurses in charge, he can never be in a command position. If he wants to make a patient feel comfortable, to regain his confidence, the doctor should be the one to put his hand in the wound or even (as I saw one of my teachers do) spoon out a fecaloma whose stench drove the nurses away.

The doctor who has mastered his art should be all these things, but to an even more complex degree. He does not face an intelligent opponent, but rather nature, which is largely unpredictable. And he is not asked to wage battle two or three times a year, but several times a day. To have the best results, he must make the best possible assessment of probabilities, referring to written records, to what he knows that has never been written down, to what he senses. He needs to have forged a valid scale of preferences and utilities. He must not be mistaken in his calculation of the risks, his decision as to how far a case can be taken.

Charity, logic, intuition, knowledge: we cultivate all of these all of our lives. As with any artists, a gift is not enough. There is also the need for the passage of time, the gradual buildup of thought and memory, the mind's work on accumulated data. It is sometimes estimated that psychoanalysis takes about one thousand hours. A pilot is considered experienced after a thousand hours of flight time. It takes about a thousand hours of judo (a longtime hobby of mine) to win a black belt.

But one of my friends, a top-level mountain climber, has already put in twenty thousand hours on the slopes. And a full-time department head in a hospital, dividing his time between practicing, teaching, and research, has devoted about one hundred thousand hours to medicine by the time he turns fifty.

I have often been impressed and attracted by young doctors with their well-organized knowledge, their eagerness to care for the sick. But the art of medicine, if it appears at all, is hard to discern before a doctor has had one hundred thousand hours of practice. It is a crying shame to force doctors who have attained this high level of competence to retire, when they could still be teaching, caring for patients, and showing through their example just what medicine is. Would anyone have dreamed of making Picasso stop painting at seventy? That is what happened to some of my teachers who were still full of energy and at the peak of their careers. They showed me what it means to be at the height of one's artistic powers, even if they were dealing with scientific data related to pharmacology, pathology, biochemistry or whatever. The notion of eliminating art from medical endeavor, making it a purely scientific pursuit, is unrealistic. On the one hand, because there will always be a degree of uncertainty requiring strategic calculation and assessment. On the other, because of the privileged relationship between strategist and patient, dependent on the necessarily nonrational trust that everything is for the best.

This is our profession's not unreasonable approach to the sublime. It can sometimes be attained, even as administrators and government officials are suggesting it should be no more than a business, complete with advertising and competition.

I have always thought that artists have a great advantage over scientists. They can capture a vision of beauty and truth, and for centuries to come their work remains unchanged. The scientist, however, approaches truth only obliquely and constantly sees his work being questioned, reshaped, placed in a different perspective, and reinterpreted, if it is not simply forgotten.

The physician's art proceeds from the same source as the painter's flash of intuition, the sculptor's skill, or the playwright's psychological powers, yet it leaves behind only the fleeting memory in the minds of the few people who witnessed it that something great was accomplished. A life was saved when it might not have been, or the will to live revived when it had been overwhelmed by anxiety, or an unwitting death sentence overturned.

It is now possible to "improve" the art of medicine by identifying gifted individuals, making therapeutic choices more rational, paying fresh attention to finalities. This is a new situation in the history of medicine, perhaps in human history. The result of parallel developments in science and humanism, it is characteristic of what we call Western civilization. It is an opportunity to reproclaim values now endangered in some cultures, but which every human being rediscovers as basic when he is near death, or thinks he is. And in this respect I was not a little impressed, I admit, to read in the works of Philo of Alexandria (c. 20 B.C.–A.D. c. 50) that a Jewish sect living along the Nile some 4,000 years ago called itself the Therapists.

In closing, I wish to offer these remarks as a tribute to all the mathematicians and ethicists I have cited. Their work, conceptual daring and intellectual courage restore medicine to its noble status at a time when it is being questioned by a troubled society. I salute doctors who are plagued by doubts, who lose sleep over difficult cases, who are crushed when they lose a patient and content to be alive when they save one. I ask those close to them to bear with them. As everyone knows, the life of an artist is not an easy one.

Bibliography

d'Aumale, Geoffroy. *La Programmation des décisions.* P.U.F. 1968, Paris.

Ballantine, H. Thomas, Jr. "Annual discourse: The crisis in ethics, anno domini 1979." *The New England Journal of Medicine,* 1979, 301, 634–638.

Batteau, Pierre, and Jean-Pierre Marciano. *Probabilités et décisions dans l'incertain.* P.U.F. 1976, Paris.

Brunel, D. *Les Mathématiques modernes, technique de décision, 2: recherche de l'optimum.* 1970, Bibliothèque d'Économie.

Chapman, Carleton B. "On the definition of teaching of the medical ethic." *The New England Journal of Medicine,* 1979, 301, 630–634.

de Jouvenel, Bertrand. *l'Art de la conjecture.* J.E.I.D.E.I.S., 1972, Paris.

Kassirer, Jerome P. "The principles of clinical decision-making: An introduction to decision analysis." *The Yale Journal of Biology and Medicine,* 1976, 49, 149–164.

Moulin, Hervé. *Théorie des jeux et sciences sociales.* La Recherche, 1978, 989, 449–456.

Niven, Ivan. *Premières notions de probabilité et analyse combinatoire.* "Les mathématiques du choix," Dunod, 1970, Paris.

Rameau, Claude. *La Prise de décision, acte de management.* Les éditions d'organisation, 1977, Paris.

Robbins, Galen, and David Wilson. *Cardiovascular clinic cueoriented computer-assisted medical record, algorithmic disease management and surveillance programs.* Health Communications and Informatics, 1979, 5, 93–100.

Saint-Sernin, Bertrand. *Les Mathématiques de la décision.* P.U.F. 1973, Paris.

Sfez, Lucien. *Critique de la décision.* Presses de la Fondation nationale des Sciences politiques, 1976, Paris.

About the Author

LUCIEN ISRAËL is head of the Hôpital Franco-Musulman in Bobigny, France, and is one of the few Europeans who is associated with the National Cancer Institute of the United States. He began his work as a pulmonary specialist and later became an oncologist.